An Introduction to Cognitive Optometry

2007

by

Nazir Brelvi, OD

Bloomington, IN  Milton Keynes, UK

authorHOUSE™

AuthorHouse™
1663 Liberty Drive, Suite 200
Bloomington, IN 47403
www.authorhouse.com
Phone: 1-800-839-8640

AuthorHouse™ UK Ltd.
500 Avebury Boulevard
Central Milton Keynes, MK9 2BE
www.authorhouse.co.uk
Phone: 08001974150

First published by AuthorHouse 5/23/2007

ISBN: 978-1-4343-0453-7 (e)
ISBN: 978-1-4343-0452-0 (sc)

Library of Congress Control Number: 2007903138

Printed in the United States of America
Bloomington, Indiana

This book is printed on acid-free paper.

Dedicated to Asjad, my "autistic" nephew,

and others like him, who are "locked"

within the confines of a neural cage.

Acknowledgements

Writing a book like this depends upon the cogitations of a large number of scientists and professional researchers, who have blazed the *neurological* trail before me. While all these sources of information are mentioned in the text or brief bibliography, I would like to acknowledge a select few that have been especially influential in helping me develop some of my ideas about the complex process of human cognition.

They are, in random order:

Christof Koch, Susan Blackmore, Vilayanur Ramachandran, Roger Penrose, Brian Josephson, John Wheeler, Steven Weinberg, Gerald Edelman, Brian Goodwin, William James, Charles Darwin, Daniel Dennett, Bernard Baars, Steven Pinker, David Bohm, Michael Gazzaniga, Allan Hobson, Ray Jackendoff, Marvin Minsky, Thomas Nagel, Satyendra Nath Bose, John Searle and Semir Zeki.

I am also indebted to my wife, Sarah, for not rolling her eyes at some of my pontifications, to Steve Kirchuk of Computer Images Web, for doing an excellent job on the illustrations and for the entire staff at AuthorHouse, especially Jennifer Handy and Kathleen, for making this book so visually pleasing.

Thank You.

"Creating a new theory is not like destroying an old barn and erecting a skyscraper in its place. It is rather like climbing a mountain; gaining new and wider views, discovering unexpected connections between our starting point and its rich environment.

But the point from which we started out still exists and can be seen, although it appears smaller and forms a tiny part of our broad view gained by our mastery of the obstacles on our adventurous way up."

Albert Einstein

Preface

Since the early dawn of prehistory, people of every known human society have sought to understand and create an orderly world around them. This constant yearning to know and derive *rationales* for our mundane existence on this Earth has provided a receptive audience for scholars, scientists and 'experts' of every persuasion.

In the past, our ancestors believed that the world around them had magical powers. They thought that angels and demons operating in mysterious ways occupied a *netherworld* of a miraculous and supernatural dimension.

Today, fewer and fewer of us believe in such a world.

For many, our existence has gradually come to be defined by nefarious politics, dubious international policies and the "hollywoodization" of popular scientific discoveries. As members of a complex society, we labor under the delusion that the ultimate goal of modern scientific endeavor is an understandable, clear and consistent model of the physical world, which would lead some day to a greater insight into the deeper mysteries of the Universe.

However, this may be fiction.

In my opinion, all we can ever hope to derive, is what the Germans call *Zeitgeist*, a self-consistent *myth* for our times. All the scientific and mathematical models, formulated by the 'educated' brethren of our learned community, may turn out to be mere *fairy* tales. For any scientific 'model' of the Universe not consistent with the sensory *repertoire* of our nervous system may be just *figments* of the imaginative human mind.

Soon after the emergence of *agrarian* cultures in the Fertile Crescent and Mesopotamia, our ancestors began to pursue pastimes that were more "cerebral". Their initial attempts to understand the surroundings and put into prose the inherent comedies or tragedies of social interaction, are evident in the musings of ancient Greek and Roman writers of yesterday.

However, even though "armchair" philosophy does produce fascinating conjecture and abstract surmise, in order to fully understand how biological systems work, increasingly innovative experiments need to be devised and the findings jotted down. Then wielding Occam's razor, the various "theories" of the mind promulgated by cognitive psychologists need to be surgically "culled", in order to lay bare the basic *tenets* of brain science and cognition.

For philosophically speaking, the central question has always been: Who are we and what does it mean to be human?

These queries initiate a discussion of the mind since mental phenomena form a bridge by which we *connect* to the rest of the world. By delving deeper, we realize that any scientific discipline dealing with human cognition requires a solid foundation in the philosophy of mind.

The rapidly emerging field of Cognitive Neuroscience will attempt to address what constitutes human reality and how it relates to Universal Reality, if there is such an entity.

It was not until the mid-17th century, after the publication of Rene Descartes' *Traite de l'homme*, where he distinguished between the *res extensa* (physical substance) and *res cogitans* (thinking substance) that philosophers and neuroscientists began to ponder in earnest the so-called mind-body duality in its present form.

However, it was Hermann von *Helmholtz*, of *Geometric Optics* fame, that contributed hugely to the early study of the nervous system. In fact, he was the first 'neuroscientist' to suggest that *invertebrates* would be good models for interpreting *vertebrate* neurology.

Starting in the 1930s, brain researchers began to discover the presence of motor and sensory "maps" in the brain. It soon became clear that *each* sensory modality had several "copies" of these maps, each mediating the local *topography* of objects recognized by the individual in the visual field.

In the 1970s and 80s, they found these multiple maps reached an incredibly high level of complexity in the primate visual system. To date, more than 30 such maps pertaining to visual information have been isolated; some uniquely specialized to subserve functions like motion, color and depth perception.

As most of us are well aware, research and development in the numerous areas of the Biological Sciences today is an enormous enterprise. Each sub-discipline sports its own gatekeepers that are loath to let "strangers" sit in on their parochial debates. Even though numerous neuroscientists have begun to piece together the intricate workings of neural networks embedded in our brains, I feel that the abilities of such neuronal coalitions to learn, reason and interact with their environment is routinely underestimated.

Instead of continuing to study the mechanical workings of neurons *ad nauseum*, we as cognitive scientists should be looking at the *global* aspects of the central nervous system (CNS). For just as an automobile is somehow, more than the sum of its parts, teasing apart its components and scrutinizing them individually in the lab, will not reveal its secrets.

As full-blooded Americans steeped in the muscle-car culture of yesteryears, we understand that in order to fully appreciate the joys of driving a well-engineered automobile, all one needs to do is "open-it-up" on the *autobahns* or cruise down US 1 with the top down.

Merely understanding the material basis of thinking or cognition is unlikely to open wide the doors of discovery. What is needed instead is a much deeper appreciation of how the sensory information gathered from the environment by our complex senses is seamlessly integrated into *cognitive* perception.

Any sound scientific theory should, based on the infamous *Occam's Rule* i.e. be able to describe a large range of natural phenomena via a few key postulates. If the predictions agree with the observations, we look further. If not, as Einstein observes at the beginning of this book, we either modify or discard the theory and start anew.

Currently, perceptual neuroscience has been able to construct reasonably sophisticated computational models to explain the neurological basis of various visual phenomena. Through the analysis of visual information processing at the retina, thalamus, brainstem, cerebral cortex and the limbic system on a global scale, we shall isolate a few of the common mechanisms used by the brain to comprehend its surroundings.

Then, integrating the sensory information harvested from the other modalities of olfaction, hearing, touch and internal awareness to the rapidity of visual processing will lead us to a fuller appreciation of human cognition.

Dr. Nazir Brelvi

Allamuchy, NJ

2007

The Brain Sciences & Optometry

Current research on neurological patients displaying a bewildering array of cognitive dysfunctions, ranging from savants to autism, has been booming over the past two decades. However, the Optometric or Vision scientists have been slow to capitalize on such emerging disciplines, and failed to "weigh-in" with their own *model* of Cognition.

The shifting paradigms of cognitive sciences have begun to provide us with a tool-kit, if you will, for making increasingly sophisticated analyses of the behavioral and/or visual deficits observed after head trauma or brain injury. Computerized neuro-imaging methods such as CT and MRI that can precisely localize brain injury *in vivo* are enabling scientists to identify and map standardized models for compromised neural pathways.

The frontiers of scientific discovery are defined as much by the tools available for observation as by conceptual innovation. Optometrists or Optometric physicians have historically studied the visual system *in toto* along with the subtle nuances associated with a plethora of learning disabilities.

The time is now ripe for Optometry to *broaden* its scientific horizons and venture into the *Brain* Sciences. Cognitive Optometry can provide a complementary view of the central role played by the visual system in the complex process of cognitive perception.

Investigating the subtle nuances of sight has several advantages over studying some of our other senses because, as humans, we are highly visual creatures. This is reflected in the large amount of brain tissue dedicated to the analysis of images and the prominence of binocularity in correctly interpreting what you see out there. Our visual percepts are vivid and rich in information.

The neuronal basis of many visual phenomena has been investigated throughout the animal kingdom. Perceptual neuroscience has advanced to such a point that reasonably sophisticated computational models have been constructed to better understand the physical basis of cognition and sentience in the brain. The real power of these tools though is still constrained by the types of problems one formulates and thus chooses to investigate.

According to Christof Koch, a pioneer brain researcher at Caltech, Pasadena and a close associate of Sir Francis Crick (the eminent co-discoverer of DNA), all the different aspects of consciousness (smell, pain, vision, touch or hearing) employ one or perhaps a few *common* mechanisms. He feels that figuring out the neuronal basis for even one of these modalities will pave the way for understanding all of them.

From an introspective point of view, this hypothesis sounds quite radical. After all, what do sounds, sights and touch have in common? Intuitively, we note that these sensory modalities mediate quite different sensations and provide insights into seemingly different worlds. Yet, current scientific research utilizing sophisticated imaging techniques reveal that similar neuronal events or circuits in the CNS, in all probability, mediate all three of these subjective sensations or *qualia*.

What still remains to be discovered are the neuronal substrates of cognition (NSC), for whenever information is represented in the NSC, one becomes subjectively conscious of it. There is, of course, the underlying assumption that consciousness depends on what is going on inside the head and not necessarily on the way the animal is behaving i.e. there is an *explicit* correspondence between any mental event and its neuronal correlates.

In other words, any change in a subjective state must be associated with a change in its neuronal state. This search for the minimal set of neuronal events/mechanisms, jointly sufficient for a specific *conscious* percept is the Holy Grail of Cognitive Neuroscience.

The allied discipline of Cognitive Optometry, however, is not so much interested in psychological labels pertaining to whether we are conscious, self-conscious or non-conscious *zombies*, safely ensconced in an elaborate

Cartesian Theater of the Mind. The broader field of Optometry has always sought to mainstream its patients by not only treating but also managing the multifaceted ramifications of binocular dysfunction.

As optometric physicians, we serve as the primary vision "gatekeepers". We evaluate patients grappling with fixation disparities, attentional deficits, perceptual anomalies, learning disabilities, language disorders and dysfunctions related to the "abnormal" processing of multimodal sensory information.

Such cognitive malfunctions, apart from being grounded in emotion and affective disorders, may also involve multifarious deficits of the visual system, aniseikonias, amblyopias and embedded refractive errors.

By introducing the emerging discipline of Cognitive Optometry, I envision our ability, as primary eyecare providers, to recognize the key role played by the visual system in the complex process of cognition.

What will mark Cognitive Optometry as a *new* discipline is the study of anomalous mental activity as a visual information-processing problem. It rests on the assumption that our perceptions, thoughts and social behavior depend on the ability of the visual system to evaluate and collate sensory information correctly.

By "translating" perceptual representations taking place in various regions of the brain into successful goal-oriented behavior we can help our debilitated patients lead more productive and rewarding lives.

Contents

Section 3 An Overview of Cognition

Section 1

Sensory Systems: An Overview

Sensory Receptors

Sensory impulses from nearly all regions of the organism's physical body are transmitted to its CNS conveying relevant information about the environment and how the organism is itself reacting to it. The anatomical structures where these sensory impulses originate are called sense organs or receptors. The main task of such receptor organs is to respond to stimuli of various kinds and intensities. In a process called transduction the receptors help "translate" the stimulus to a language easily understood and "spoken" by the neurons of the nervous system i.e. convert electrical impulses into action potentials.

The stimulus alters the permeability of the receptor membrane, usually by opening the sodium (Na^+) channels and thus depolarizing the receptor. The act of depolarization sets up a graded change in the membrane potential in a process similar to the synaptic activation of a neuron. The mechanism behind transduction is not fully understood in its entirety especially when the action potentials lead to a subjective construct or "feeling" in the brain.

Most receptors are built to respond only or preferentially to one kind of stimulus energy, be it mechanical, chemical, thermal or visual. The kind of stimulus to which the receptor responds most easily is called an *adequate* stimulus. However, most receptors are able to respond to stimuli of other kinds (inadequate stimuli) although the threshold for activation or evoking a response may be slightly higher. We shall explore this built-in capability of receptors in our discussion of *synesthesia* and *blindsight* in later sections.

Since only humans are able to inform the observer directly of what they feel, animal experiments alone cannot resolve the question of the relationship between receptors and conscious sensations. Not all impulses reaching the CNS from the receptors are consciously perceived for a considerable "editing", if you will, exists at all levels of sensory pathway integration to censor "irrelevant" information and enhance "relevant" ones. This property of the CNS implies that the receptors do not provide the brain with an objective or true representation of its surroundings.

Modern neuroscientists are still unable to explain how action potentials, which are very similar in all nerve fibers, are able to evoke dissimilar conscious sensations in different individuals. They have theorized that the brain has a built-in ability to *collate* disparate bits and pieces of all relevant sensory information into a coherent and unified percept of the world out there to give it meaning.

A single neuron's membership in any neural network mediating sensory information is probably fluid and may change from moment to moment when it interacts with several such networks in its vicinity. In addition, the neuron's firing cadence may also be modulated by the animal's past perceptual experiences, its internal brain dynamics (whether it is actively or passively sampling its immediate environment) and the animal's expectations for the future.

Brain scientists now believe that the final processing depends on the extensive interconnections found among cortical areas mediating various aspects of sensory information. These specialized areas, found to be clustered in the forehead region of the skull, then interpret which "messages" are being conveyed, assigns a priority status to them and "decide" how the particular individual should respond.

Evolution of the Nervous System

The nervous system is the most complex of all the organ systems in the animal embryo. Billions of nerve cells or neurons develop a highly organized pattern of connections, creating the neuronal network that makes up the functioning brain and the rest of the nervous system.

There are many hundreds of different types of neurons, differing in identity and connectivity even though they may appear quite similar. There are also supporting tissues in the nervous system, known collectively as glia; for example, Schwann cells surround the axons of peripheral neurons whereas oligodendrocytes and astrocytes ensheath the central neurons.

All nervous systems, vertebrate and invertebrate, provide a system of communication through this highly anastomotic network of nerve cells comprising various shapes and sizes. Each neuron connects with its target cell at synapses, sites at which the propagation of an action potential induces neurotransmitter release. The nervous system can only function properly if the neurons correctly connect to one another and thus a central question surrounding the CNS development is how various neurons connect with such preciseness and specificity.

Specific chemicals acted as intercellular transmitters in the developing zygote's homeostatic system and various chemical messengers housed in its plasma membrane, regulated and controlled its day-to-day activities via these molecular interactions. As the organism became multi-cellular, this 'local' interaction was expanded to reach other component cells, whose activities were also regulated and coordinated for maximum efficiency.

The centralized nervous system with its constituent neurons communicated with each other or with effector organs via chemical agents known as neurotransmitters. Here one neuron alters the activity of the next neuron in a reflex chain by releasing a specific chemical messenger, which diffuses across a very narrow gap (synapse). One important characteristic of chemical mediation that is understandable in terms of membrane receptors is specificity.

A chemical messenger – hormone, neurotransmitter or locally released *paracrine* – influences only certain cells and not others. The explanation is that the membranes or cytoplasm of different cell types, differ in the types of receptors they contain. A single cell usually contains many different receptor types, each capable of combining with only one chemical messenger. In addition, the receptors themselves are subject to physiological regulation i.e. the number and affinity of the receptors to their specific chemical messenger can be increased or decreased, through a mechanism of feedback control.

How does the messenger-receptor combination elicit the cell's responses?

It usually gets quite complicated and requires the participation of so-called *second messengers*. These are substances generated within the cell or that enter its cytosol via mediated transport. This messenger then triggers the cell's overall response. The same ones may operate in many areas of the body and in different types of cells.

The two best understood second messengers at present are calcium and cyclic AMP (cAMP). Both may sometimes be involved in eliciting the cell's response in the same situation. Also, just because the researchers have isolated calcium and cAMP as *second messengers*, does not mean that these are the only possible ones. Others almost certainly remain to be discovered.

Since the CNS was not designed by some supernatural agency or intrepid engineer, but emerged through the relentless process of natural selection, over immense *eons* of time, neural variability is a fundamental property of the CNS found in any specified animal population. Natural selection, of course, is not the *only* process that modifies organisms or their nervous systems over generations but so far it is seems to be the only known process in nature that appears to *design* them.

During the early stages of evolution, the 'nervous' system was very simple. It 'orientated' the organism within its habitat by mediating movement. In case of the bacterial cell, it propelled the organism towards or away from a source of stimulation, depending on whether it indicated the presence of friend or foe, food or poison. The response was essentially *chemotactic* in nature.

Soon, these membrane receptors, arrayed on the outer surface of the organism, began to involute as the organism became multicellular and multi-layered. They took on the appearance of the synaptic terminals, simple ionic 'gates' initially and evolving into the more complex ones seen today in higher animals.

Next, a more amplified version of a 'truer' nervous system was wrought, with a limited number of interneurons interposed between the afferent and efferent nerve cells. The interneuronal component then began to expand rapidly until it came to be by far the largest part. The interneurons formed smaller 'networks' of increasing complexity, as the housekeeping chores of the organism increased.

At first, the nervous system mediated mainly the stability of the internal environment and position of the body in 3D space. These cells then, with increasing specialization of function, came to be localized at the business *end* of the primitive nervous system. As the organisms became bilaterally symmetrical, the sense organs migrated to the site of the *stoma* or mouth, giving rise to the brain and cranial nerves around it.

According to Stuart Kaufmann, a proponent of Complexity Theory that looks for mathematical principles of order underlying many complex systems in the universe like meteorological phenomena, human societies, crystal formation, galaxies, brain formation etc., such feats of self-organization, order, stability and coherence may be an innate property of some complex systems. "Evolution," he suggests, "may be a marriage of natural selection and self-organization."

His theory does raise some interesting issues. Natural selection presupposes that a "replicator" arose somehow that allowed an organism to react to the vagaries of nature by undergoing mutations for traits that would enhance its coping ability. Kaufmann asserts that for evolution to occur at all, mutations have to modify a physical body enough to make a difference in its functioning but not so much that it will incapacitate the creature. The process of natural selection would have to work within the constraints of these principles just at it works within the biological ones that define living things.

We tend to view brain evolution as *additive* rather than nonlinear i.e. the complex human brain is simply an ape brain with a few 'new' parts added. In actuality, we should visualize our brain as a unique amalgamation of evolutionary old and newer areas that have been honed and modified to successfully adapt human behavior to the challenges of environmental demands.

Steven Pinker in his recent, euphemistically titled tome: *How the Mind Works*, observes..."the fallacy that intelligence is some exalted ambition of evolution is part of the same fallacy that treats it as a divine essence or wonder tissue or all-compassing mathematical principle. The mind is an organ, a biological gadget. We have our minds because their design attains outcomes whose benefits outweighed the costs in the lives of Plio-Pleistocene African primates."

Evolutionary psychologists do not believe that all behaviors are driven by genetic mechanisms. They think that the brain has built-in adaptations, which are of a more general nature. These adaptations are a set of rules that govern our behavior. Moreover, since there are an infinite number of environments, these rules apply differently in each situation, resulting in an infinite number of behaviors.

In fact, a major assumption in the biological sciences is under siege: the idea that a larger brain with more cells is responsible for the greater computational capacity observed in the *Homo* lineage. Numerous studies and accumulating neurological data show that the human brain's unique abilities are not a function of cell number but the emergence of specialized circuitry.

Split-brain studies, where the corpus callosum is severed leaving behind two isolated 600-650 gm brains rather than just one 1200 gm organ point out that the capacity of the left half (the size of a chimp brain) remains unchanged from its preoperative human level.

Many lines of anatomical and physiological research have found that there are indeed specializations in human brain tissue. The physiological properties of dendritic spines differ from those of other primates. The primary and secondary visual, somatosensory and auditory cortices express varying distributions of specific nerve fibers and the density of certain nerve cells called *chandelier* cells differ between prefrontal and visual cortical regions.

The nonhuman primate and human visual systems also have different organizational properties. When comparing, for example, the anterior commissure between the macaque and humans, the monkeys are still able to process visual information through it when the corpus callosum is severed whereas humans cannot. Lesions to V1 in humans cause blindness whereas monkeys with similar lesions are still capable of residual vision.

Other examples also abound of system-level variations between primates and humans even though both visual systems have virtually identical sensory capacities.

Development of the Nervous System

The gradual maturation of the CNS is easily observed first-hand in the puzzling phenomenon of embryogenesis, when the unicellular zygote undergoes a breathtaking transformation from an amoeba-like single cell to a multi-cellular mammalian species, during the course of a single pregnancy. While the eggs of vertebrates differ greatly in size and character, all the embryos pass through a stage of development where they appear somewhat similar.

How neurons assemble into discrete nuclei and how these in turn interconnect is largely determined genetically: our genes contain the "recipe" for the building of the nervous system in considerable detail. Therefore, each individual neuron possesses the instructions that determine its final size, the shape of its dendritic tree and the types of neurotransmitters it uses. However, the normal development and maturation of a specific neuron is also influenced to a large degree by its neighboring cells and their interconnections i.e. both nature and nurture play a vital role in the final architecture of the mature organism.

A few days after fertilization, the intricate process of cell differentiation transforms the *morula* (cluster of embryonic cells into a mulberry-like mass) into an elongated disc. In the third week (after 18 days), the development of the nervous system begins in earnest with the formation of a *neural plate* in the prospective cranial end of the disc.

In a process called *neurulation*, the main body axis forms and the various layers of tissue become well defined. The neural tube and notochord (a stiff rod of cells forming the 'back-bone') emerge and the tube differentiates into the brain and spinal cord. The brain section subdivides into the forebrain, midbrain and hindbrain, which later on give rise to the specialized 'association' areas of the cortex that mediate all voluntary and involuntary activities.

Various so-called *tool-kit* genes for constructing three-dimensional structures are activated, which begin laying down the building blocks of vertebrate brains. The control of individual tool-kit gene action and anatomy is done via numerous *genetic switches* that encode instructions unique to specific species.

These are lengthy sequences of DNA, bound by a variety of proteins, that transform complex sets of inputs into simpler outputs; analogous to a work order in an assembly plant that breaks down the building of a complex machine into simple operations at various stations. Many separate switches may regulate one gene such that it ends up being used numerous times and in different locations.

In the fourth week, three swellings or primary vesicles take shape. The cavity within these pouches is continuous and develops into the ventricular system of the adult brain. The ependymal cells lining the inner wall of the ventricles produce copious amounts of CSF, which now fills it up. The most cranial vesicle forms the forebrain, the middle one gives rise to the midbrain structures and the caudal-most evolves into the hindbrain.

Early in the fourth week, the ventral aspect of the neural tube exhibits shallow, transverse grooves (branchial arches). They represent the first segregation of neurons that later differentiate into the various nuclei of the brainstem. Thus, several cranial nerves and their nuclei are initially laid down in segments corresponding to the *gill arches* of the primordial vertebrate body plan.

The simple layering of the neural tube, with the mantle zone (gray matter) inside and the marginal zone (white matter) outside is retained in the spinal cord. In the cranial part of the neural tube (the future brain), however, major alterations in the mutual positions of these occur forming a layered sheet of gray matter externally just under the pia.

Also in the fourth week, a shallow furrow, the *sulcus limitans*, at the lower limit of the brainstem, marks the border between the *basal* plates (source of motor neurons) and the *alar* plates (give rise to the sensory neurons). This corresponds to the functional division between the ventral and dorsal *horns* of the spinal cord. In the adult brainstem, the *sulcus limitans* delineates the motor and sensory cranial nerve nuclei. Several neuronal groups in the brainstem migrate from their birthplace in the alar or basal plates.

The cerebral hemispheres begin to form in the fifth week along with the basal ganglia and the internal capsule. As development proceeds, the caudate nucleus and the thalamus come to lie medial to the internal capsule whereas the lentiform nucleus (globus pallidus and putamen) lie laterally.

At the beginning of the eighth week, neuroblasts from the mantle zone migrate into the marginal zone to establish the cerebral cortex. The differentiation from the cortical plate to the six-layered cortex is not complete until after birth and is accomplished by waves of cells migrating toward the cortical surface. Since the deeper layers are laid down first, the neurons destined for the more superficial ones have to "surf" through them guided by the processes of radially oriented glial cells extending from the ependyma to the pia.

Postnatally, several serial but temporally overlapping processes mark development. There is a continuation of synaptogenesis, which begins prior to birth and in humans occurs at different rates in different brain regions. Synapses in the brain begin to form much before birth, prior to week 27 (counting from conception) in humans, but do not reach peak density for 15 months after birth.

Synaptogenesis is more pronounced early on in the deeper cortical layers and occurs later in the more superficial layers. The neurons are also increasing the size of their dendritic arborizations now, extending their axons and undergoing vigorous myelination. Synaptogenesis is followed by synaptic pruning, which continues for more than a decade. This pruning allows the CNS to fine-tune neural connectivity. For instance, the ocular dominance columns in the visual cortex initially show a much larger overlap between the projections of the two eyes onto neurons in V1 than after the pruning is complete.

There is compelling evidence that different regions of the human brain reach maturity at different times. For instance, synapses in the superior temporal region of the auditory cortex, reach peak density earlier in postnatal development (age 3 months), than those in the association cortex of the frontal lobes (age 15 months). Some data also suggest that in humans, the processes of synaptogenesis and synaptic pruning follow different time courses in sensory and motor cortices than the association cortices. Such heterogeneous developmental changes correlate with the developmental time courses observed by Jean Piaget.

The human brain undergoes changes until the late teens, when in most respects it resembles the adult brain. Throughout adulthood, it changes very little in terms of volume, myelination and synaptic density until well into the seventh decade of life, when some reductions in brain volume are seen due to attritional neuronal loss. Yet, recent evidence reveals that new neurons may well be produced throughout adulthood.

Individual neurons can inform others about the strength of the stimulus it receives, such as the intensity of the impinging sound or light waves by varying the frequency and pattern of its firing rate. It seems to be using a frequency code, if you will, to communicate or broadcast its level of stimulation. Even though the firing frequencies vary with different classes of neurons, some are capable of achieving rates in excess of 100 Hz per second.

Burst neurons produce trains of action potentials with an intermittent pattern of high frequency discharges, while the single spike ones fire at intervals that are more regular. Others can switch between these two modes depending on which neurotransmitter acts as the triggering agent. Serotonin tends to evoke *plateau* potentials in groups of spinal motoneurons, which play a prominent role in mediating attention or motivation behaviors rather than transmit specific information.

Overall, the code for the information carried by an axon in the human retina is the frequency and pattern of action potentials its cells generate since the strength of action potential is always the same.

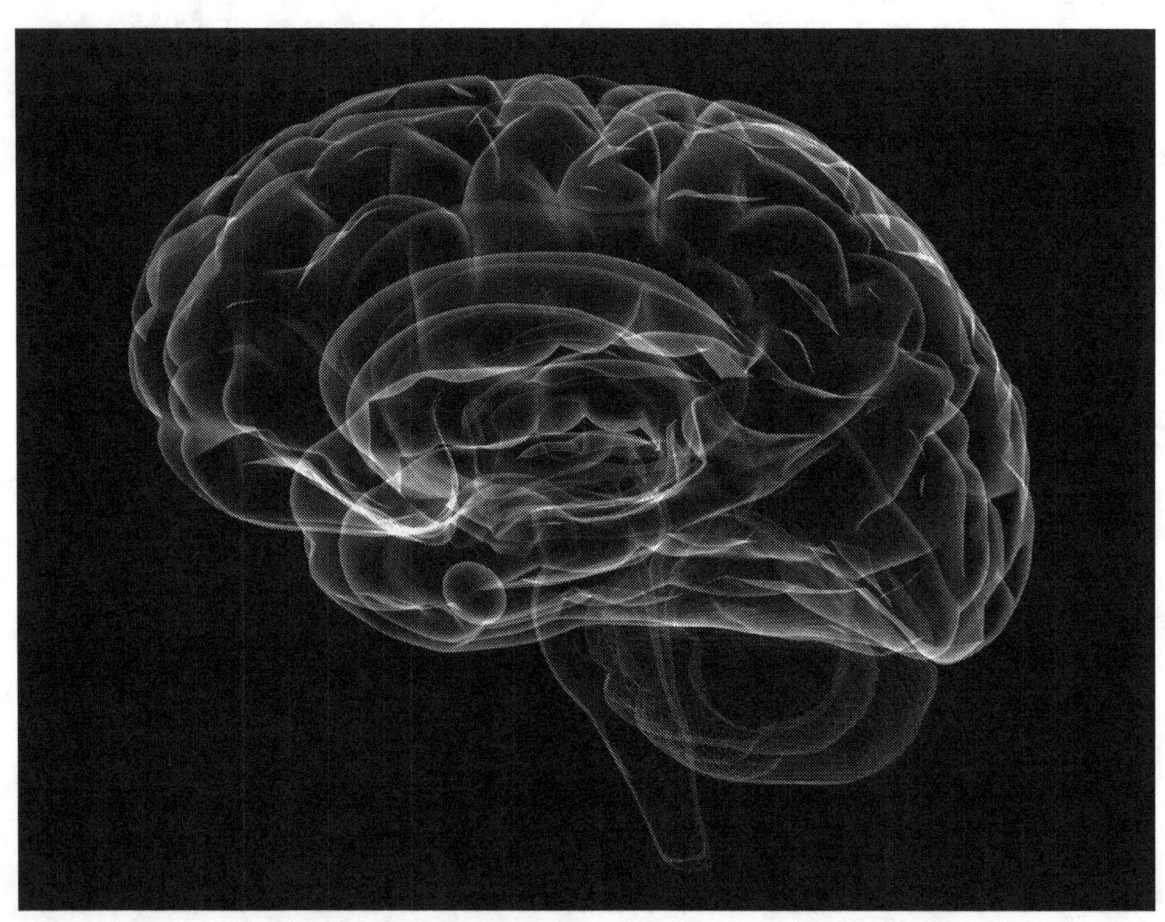

MRI scan depicting Gross Anatomy of the Brain

Brains

Why did brains evolve anyway? Why do animals need a brain?

The short answer to this profound query is to *process* information! Most organisms in order to survive have to make choices every time they decide to move, stop, eat or explore their surroundings. In the unicelled amoeba, *putzing* around in the backyard pond, this may consist of relatively simple tasks of discovering or avoiding. In multicellular animals, these choices rest on how efficiently the information is gathered and converted into crucial decisions. The more you know, the better decisions one can make. The organism's nervous system and brain makes all this possible.

Natural selection cannot directly endow an organism with information about its environment or mental organs to process it but only choose between appropriate genes. However, genes build brains and different genes are capable of building brains that process information in diverse ways. A new field of computer science called *genetic algorithms* has shown that Darwinian selection can create increasingly intelligent software.

Genetic algorithms are programs that are duplicated to make multiple copies, though with random mutations that makes each one a tiny bit different. All copies then have a go at solving a problem and the ones that do best are allowed to reproduce to furnish the copies for the next round.

But first, parts of each program are randomly mutated again, split in two and the halves exchanged. After many cycles of computation, selection, mutation and reproduction, the surviving programs are found to be better than any a human programmer could have designed.

More apropos of how a mind can evolve, genetic algorithms have been applied to various neural networks participating in a so-called robotic 'thought experiment'. A given network has inputs from simulated sense organs and outputs to simulated motor systems embedded in a virtual environment with scattered 'food' items also made available to numerous other competing networks. The ones that get the most food leave the most copies prior to the next round of mutation and selection.

The 'mutations' are random changes in the connection weights, sometimes followed by 'sexual' recombination (swapping some of their connection weights) between networks. During the early iterations, the automatons wander randomly over the terrain, occasionally bumping into a food source. However, as they 'evolve', they manage to zip from one food source to another with impunity. Indeed, a population of networks that is allowed to evolve innate connection weights often does better than a single neural network left to its own devices.

This is especially true for networks with multiple hidden layers, which complex animals, including some humans, surely possess. It was found that if a certain network could only learn but not evolve, the environmental teaching signal was soon 'diluted' during its propagation back to the hidden layers. It was then only capable of nudging the connection weights up or down by tiny increments.

However, when a network population could evolve without learning, the numerous mutations and recombinations it underwent during the simulation were able to reprogram the hidden layers directly. In fact, this occurred to such an extent that the network's innate connections were fine-tuned to an optimum configuration. The *geeks* found that its innate structure was selected for.

Evolution and learning can also go on simultaneously with the innate structure evolving in an animal that also learns. A population of networks can be equipped with a generic learning algorithm and can be allowed to evolve the innate parts that the network designer would ordinarily have built in by guesswork, tradition or trial-n-error.

The innate specs include how many units there are, how they are connected, what the initial connection weights are and how much the weights should be nudged up or down on each learning episode. Simulated evolution gives the networks a big head start in their learning careers.

Interestingly, James Baldwin, a psychologist from the turn of the century, had proposed that learning could also guide evolution in precisely this way, creating an illusion of Lamarckian evolution without there actually being one. Called the Baldwin Effect, it is now thought to play a key role in the evolution of brains. Contrary to traditional social science assumptions, learning is not some pinnacle of evolution attained only recently by human beings.

All but the simplest of animals are capable of learning. That is why mentally uncomplicated creatures like fruit flies and sea slugs have been convenient subjects for neuroscientists in search of the neural correlates of learning. If the ability to learn was in place in an early ancestor of multicellular animals, it could have guided the evolution of nervous systems toward their specialized circuits even when they are so intricate that natural selection could not have found them on its own.

Basic Architecture of the Brain

When the brain is viewed in a container filled with formalin in any neuro-lab, one notices that three coverings called the *dura*, the *pia* and the *arachnoid* envelope the entire brain. The *dura* is the toughest and surrounds the brain, all around and in between. The *pia* is very thin and membranous, containing most of the brain's extensive blood supply. The *arachnoid* is sandwiched between these two layers and is filled in with the cerebro-spinal fluid (CSF), which apart from other functions adds buoyancy to the brain tissue. This effectively protects the brain from being jostled around and reduces its overall weight from a robust 3 pounds to a mere 50 grams.

After the dura is peeled away, it reveals the pinkish-gray walnut-like surface split in the middle by a huge fissure. The raised rounded sections are called *gyri* and the deeper fissures or creases underlying the purplish blood vessels are known as *sulci*. A quick dissection through the hemispheres exposes some internal structures organized into white and gray matter. The gray matter forms a continuous sheet overlying a homogenous mass of white matter. The gray matter contains cell bodies of neurons and glia whereas the white matter contains the fatty myelin sheathed axons of these neurons.

The *pia* consists of an outer epipial layer and an inner membranous one called the *intima pia*. This layer invaginates, where the blood vessels enter and leave the CNS, forming a perivascular space. It derives its nutrition from the CSF and underlying neural tissue. The epipial layer consists of a meshwork of collagenous fiber bundles continuous with the *arachnoid* trabeculae. The blood vessels of the spinal cord lie within the epipial layer. The cerebral vessels lie on the surface of the Intima pia within the subarachnoid space.

In the region of the *conus medullaris*, the epipial tissue forms a covering of the *filum terminale*, fine processes of deeply located fibrous astrocytes. The CSF fills up the subarachnoid space between the delicate, non-vascular *arachnoid* and the epipial layer. Several invaginations along the deeper sulci of the brain result in a pooling of the CSF forming discrete '*cisternae*'.

The *ambiens* or superior cistern surrounds the posterior, superior and lateral surfaces of the midbrain. It is of special significance as it contains the Great Vein of Galen, the posterior cerebral, superior cerebellar arteries and the Pineal gland, adjacent to the III ventricle. CSF formed in the lateral and 3rd ventricles passes via the cerebral aqueduct into the 4th ventricle.

From there it flows out of the median and two lateral apertures into the cerebello-medullary cistern, flows out into the contiguous subarachnoid spaces of the brain and spinal cord. The bulk of the CSF returns to the venous system via the *arachnoid granulations* and *villi*. The rate of exit is pressure dependent and one-way only.

In regions adjacent to the Superior Sagittal Sinus (SSS), multiple tufted prolongations protrude through the meningeal layer of the Dura. These granulations are variable in number and location, each consisting of numerous arachnoid villi surrounded by venous lacunae. These passive one-way valves have membranes, which are readily permeable, allowing even plasma proteins and serum albumin to pass through.

The rate of CSF formation in humans is approx. 600-700 ml/day. Since the total volume of the ventricles and subarachnoid spaces is only about 140 ml in volume, the daily turnover seems to be appreciable. The CSF has a nutritive function and that it serves to remove the waste products of neuronal metabolism. The characteristic distributions of ions and non-electrolytes in the CSF and plasma imply that the CSF cannot be a simple filtrate or dialysate of the blood plasma. Current evidence supports the theory that it is a secretory product involving active transport mechanisms with expenditure of cellular energy.

Recent studies indicate extensive plexi of *serotonin* axons in the supra and sub-ependymal systems lining the walls of the ventricles and the arachnoid sheaths draping the major cerebral blood vessels originating in the *Raphe* nuclei of the Pons. These may be major modifiers of the local CSF composition and cerebral blood-flow through vascular regulation. In addition, the presence of such biogenic amines in the CSF could help mediate the release of hormones along the Hypothalamic-Pituitary axis.

The human brain represents a unique amalgamation of evolutionary older and newer areas that were modified in predictable ways. Some that underwent an expansion, some reduction, whereas others ended up wired in novel ways as the organism adapted to fresher environmental demands.

Evolutionary psychologists believe that the brain has inbuilt adaptations (a set of general rules that govern behavior) that functionally contribute to the organism's propagation. In their view, the brain does not perform any significant metabolic, mechanical or chemical service for the animal but serves a purely informational, computational or regulatory function.

A detailed mapping of these abilities is an indispensable first step in the neuroscience research enterprise. Two prominent methods are the PET (positron emission tomography) and functional MRI (fMRI). Both detect subtle changes in metabolism or blood flow in the brain while the subject is actively engaged in cognitive tasks. As such, they enable the researchers to identify brain regions that are activated during these tasks and to test hypotheses about functional brain anatomy.

The Cerebral Cortex (CC)

The comprehensive exploration of the cortex had to await the advent of modern microscopy, biochemical stains and various dyes that selectively bind to diverse cellular elements. With this enhanced ability to target specific molecular constituents of neurons, the cortex has been catalogued and mapped quite extensively.

The human cerebral cortex is very intricately organized and considered one of the most densely populated tissues in the body. It has about 30 billion neurons in total, where each cubic mm houses 100,000 neurons. Each of these neurons has upwards of 10,000 connections or synapses. No one has really made an exact count of the different types of neurons in the brain, but it could be in the neighborhood of about fifty.

One general characteristic of its operation is the astonishing variety and specificity of the actions it performs. Sensory systems handle an almost infinite variety of images, scenes, sounds, etc., which react to them in detail with remarkable accuracy. The actual body of a single neuron may measure a few tens of a micron in diameter but its axon could extend from a few mms to even a meter in length. Flanking each of these neurons is a *glial* (glue like) cell, which supports and nourishes it.

In order to better understand, consciousness as a *process* and an *emergent* property of the CNS, the reader needs to have a usable knowledge of its architecture, its anatomical organization and the remarkable dynamics it generates. The adult human brain weighs about 3 pounds and is among the most complicated objects in the universe. It is certainly one of the most remarkable biological structures to have emerged during the evolutionary process containing upwards of a 100 billion neurons.

Confronted with a structure as complex as the cortex, most scientists divide it into increasingly smaller and smaller sections in order to understand it better. A deeply held belief among biologists is that structure and function may be intimately related i.e. if any increase in the cellular density is detected or changes are noticed in the degree of myelination or certain neurological enzymes mysteriously emerge in the CSF, then it is very likely that some functional border has been broached.

Until the mid-1970's, it was widely believed that structure and function are intimately related i.e. differences in structure are reflected in differences in function and vice versa. If the cellular packing density increases or the degree of myelination changes or some enzyme makes a debut, then it is very likely that a functional border has been crossed.

Do the deep folds or grooves discernable on the outside of the cerebral hemispheres demarcate disparate regions subserving different functions? Or, are these just folds resulting from shoving a large pancake-like cortex sheet into a cramped cranial cavity? What is the exact relationship among all these areas? Do the interconnections reveal anything novel about its large-scale architecture? Are these areas randomly bunched together to fit inside the skull or is there some underlying hierarchy?

A key principle of neuronal architecture is that nearby neurons encode similar information. This widespread feature of the cortex and other nervous tissues economizes on total wiring length. Spatial clustering also shows up in different ways.

The various lobes of the CC play a diverse functional role in neural processing. Major identifiable systems can be localized within each lobe, but as we shall see some of the major systems like hearing or sight are much more widespread and highly interactive.

While all of the neocortex behind the central sulcus deals with sensory input and perception, the concern of the frontal lobes, the larger expanse of cortical matter lying forward to it is action oriented. Motor, premotor, prefrontal and anterior cingulate cortices all belong to the frontal lobes. Cognitive brain systems rely on both cortical and sub-cortical components to act as modulators of their main activities.

The frontal lobe plays a key role in the planning and execution of movements. Its two main subdivisions known as the motor contains massive clusters of neurons whose axons extend to the spinal cord and brainstem. The other, called the prefrontal, mediates the higher aspects of motor control and tasks that require the integration of information over longer time periods. Its also maintains interconnectivity with structures of the limbic lobe.

Areas of the parietal lobe receive inputs from the somato-sensory relays of the thalamus that represent information about touch, pain, temperature sense, and limb proprioception.

(Author's Note: The volume of neocortex that cannot be categorized as sensory or motor has traditionally been termed the *association* cortex. These areas receive collateral inputs from one or more modalities, which serve to provide "contextual or orientational" information in order to correct any inaccuracies in performing the task at hand.)

Numerous animal studies with microelectrodes reveal segregated cortical neighborhoods whose neurons are specialized to carry out different jobs. For example, neurons in one occipito-temporal region are especially sensitive to the hue of a certain object, whereas the ones in a region of the posterior parietal cortex mediate complex eye movements. These observations are borne out very well in human patients that present with focal deficits secondary to trauma or stroke episodes.

Cortical areas in the back of the brain, known to scientists as the visual cortex, seem to follow a 'loose' hierarchy comprising of at least a dozen levels, each subordinate to the other. When a group of neurons within one of these regions receives a strong input from a 'lower' layer, it undergoes a rapid 'weighted-average' evaluation and gets 'bumped-up' to the next 'higher' layer in the hierarchy, analogous to an irate patient's complaint being kicked-up to the entry-level employee's manager.

If the incoming information is kind of 'sketchy' or incomplete and not amenable to an unambiguous interpretation, then that particular network will 'fill-in' the deficits, arriving at a 'best guess' solution. This type of 'filling-in' occurs throughout the cortex. If the irate patient is still unhappy, the complaint rises further up the 'chain-of-command'.

The brain scientists are puzzled as to why this hierarchy exists. One reason may be that such an architecture, permits 'higher' cortical regions to 'track' *correlations* among neurons in 'lower' areas. In other words, keeping with the 'corporate' analogy, the entry-level 'lower' personnel carry on with their 'housekeeping' chores, while the 'higher' corporate executives progressively make 'broader' and 'more important' decisions.

Modern-day cognitive neurobiologists no longer describe the various nuclei and regions of the brain but instead concentrate on three major topological systems that mediate its global functioning. These are:

(1) The thalamo-cortical system, which consists of a dense meshwork of reciprocal connections between the thalamus and numerous cortical regions,

(2) a long, polysynaptic loop system organized in a set of parallel, unidirectional chains, which link the cortex to the Cerebellum, Basal ganglia and the Hippocampus, and

(3) An extensive but diffuse set of connections emanating from the Locus Coeruleus and Raphe nuclei of the brainstem and projecting out like a fan into the cerebral cortex.

The thalamus and the cortex evolved in close relationship to each other. Except for the sense of smell, all sensory modalities relay through the thalamus and on to the cortex. Neurons in the numerous thalamic nuclei fall into two broad classes: excitatory projection ones that convey impulses to the cortex and local, inhibitory interneurons.

The projection neurons are further categorized into *core* and *matrix* ones. Core cells aggregate in clusters and target *precisely delineated* recipient zones in the *intermediate* cortical layers of different regions. Matrix projection neurons reach in a more *diffuse* manner into the *superficial* layers of several *contiguous* areas of the cortex. They help disperse and synchronize the activity of literally hundreds of cells.

While all of the neocortex situated behind the central sulcus (the deep groove that partitions off the front part of each hemisphere from the back), mediates sensory input and perception, the large expanse of neocortex lying forward of it is geared for 'action'. As organisms evolve, the complexity of their actions increases and their goals extend in space and time, coming to depend less on instinctual drive and more on prior experience, insight and reasoning.

This necessitates planning, decision-making in uncertain environments, cognitive control, recall and differential diagnoses. The prefrontal cortex mediates all these so-called high-level *executive* issues. It integrates information from *all* sensory and motor modalities.

The various components of the brain function not only as individual processors of discrete signals but also 'collate' their 'graded' responses and interact with each other to produce an integrated, unified conscious response. Although the overall pattern of connections of a given brain region is describable in general terms, the microscopic variability in any human is enormous, giving it a unique signature.

Together with the morphological peculiarities of the brain and its neural connections with the body's sensory receptors, the animal is provided with a large set of constraints whose role in fostering species-specific perceptual categorization or adaptive learning cannot be underestimated.

The way in which patterns of activity in the brain change with time produces a widespread synchronization of many different functionally specialized areas, helping to integrate the sensory and motor processes. This integration ultimately gives rise to perceptual categorization, the ability to discriminate an object or event from a background for adaptive purposes.

Cognitive Neuroscience:
A Brief Historical Perspective

It seems to have all begun with Plato, the unspoken father of Western philosophy, when he declared the presence of an immortal soul imprisoned in a mortal human body. He believed that ideas have a real existence and live on forever. Most people in the West today accept some form of *dualism*. They believe they have both a mind or a soul and a body. Not surprisingly, these beliefs are widely shared by many religions and faiths all over the world, forming the basis of numerous modern philosophical perspectives.

Until the inception of experimental psychological science, the mind had been the province of philosophers, who wondered about the nature of knowledge, about how we as humans come to *know* things i.e. cognate and gain knowledge. The British philosophers, from Thomas Hobbs in the 17th century, up through John Locke and David Hume, well into the 19th century, all emphasized the role of empiricism in the production of ideas and concepts. When these interacted and coalesced, they added to an individual's knowledge system.

In 1911, Thorndike articulated his law of effect, which essentially proposed that a response that was followed by a reward would be stamped into the organism as a habitual response. If there were no reward forthcoming, the animal's response would disappear. Behaviorist psychology ruled the day and asserted that sensory information was merely data on which pre-existing mental structures acted.

Gestalt psychologists emerged and reported that percepts were best understood in relation to a stimulus's emergent properties. They existed only as a function of built-in properties of the brain. It was not learned behavior i.e. not conducive to conditioning.

It was not until well into the 1950s that cognitive awakenings began to occur, initiated in part by a now famous meeting on artificial intelligence (AI) held at Dartmouth College with Marvin Minsky, Claude Shannon and numerous well-renowned MIT celebrities in attendance. The basic tenets of what is now known, as embodied cognition were cemented in place.

(Embodied or enactive cognition are names for the general idea that a 'mind' can be created only by interacting in real time with a real environment).

I agree.

I endorse the suggestion that the mind phenomenon is an '*emergent*' property of the young CNS, found in early childhood in humans. It is 'bottom-up' in configuration and seems to be behavior-based initially. Various researchers in AI have learned that remarkably 'intelligent' behaviors can *emerge* from rather simple systems based on simple rules.

There are many examples of such emergence in biology, especially among the social insects like the honeybees, ants, termites etc. In humans, intelligence may 'coalesce' from the integration of many separate modules in the cortex. The outside world serves as its own model. No 'internal' representations are needed or seem to be necessary at the 'concept-building' stages encountered in early childhood.

As the toddler develops, his 'intelligence' begins to *evolve*, progressing from the 'behavior-based' to the more advanced 'knowledge-based' top-down kind. Inner representations of the outside world slowly coalesce and a 'know-it-all' attitude seems to emerge in the pre-teen human. Imagining, reasoning and daydreaming are now possible, which gradually merge into a more adult-like 'mindset' in the later teenage/ young adult years.

Nazir Brelvi, OD

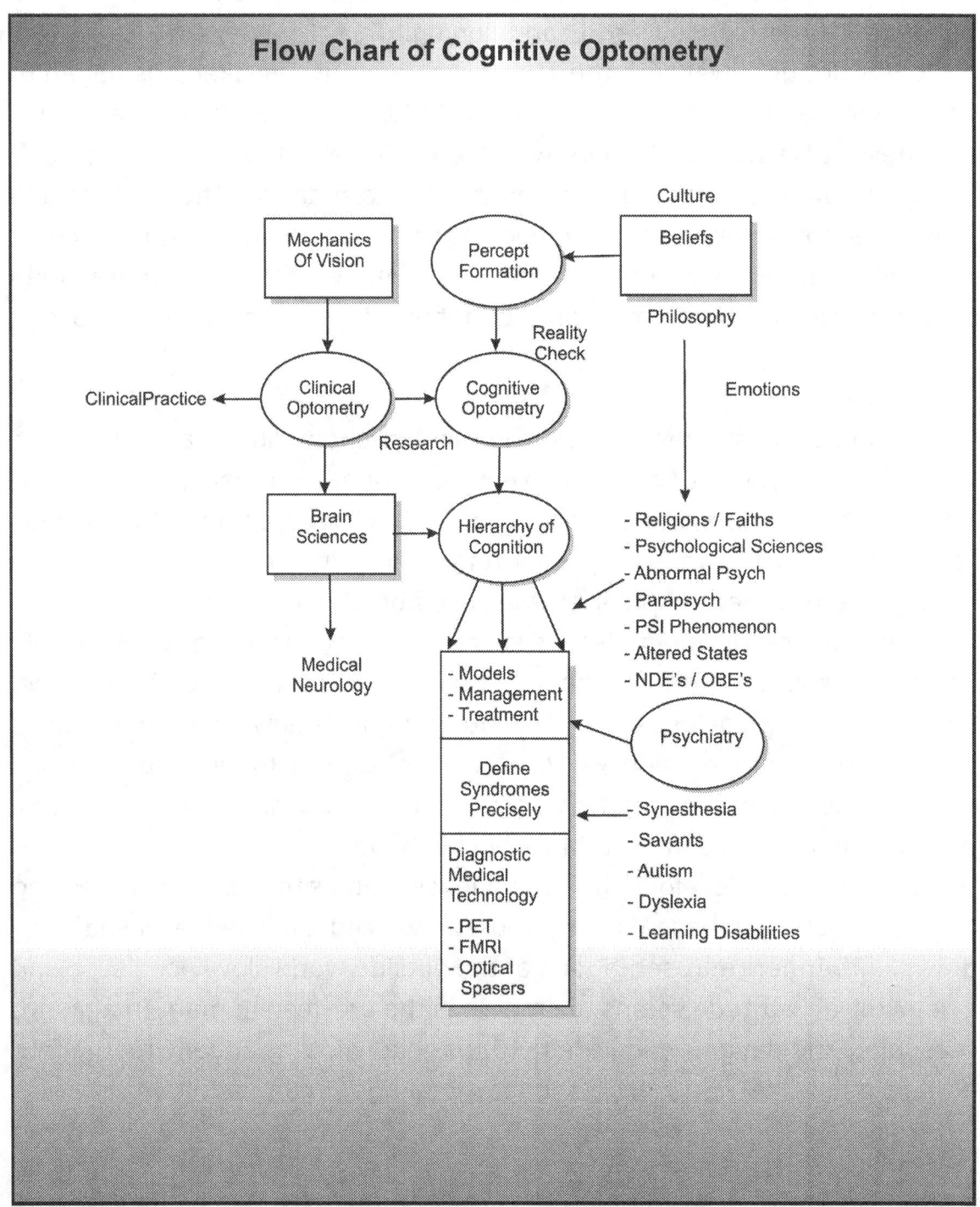

Flow Chart of Cognitive Optometry image

The term *cognitive neuroscience*, so the story goes, was coined in the grimy interior of a NYC cab as it inched down York Ave towards Rockefeller University, back in the 1970s. Neuroscientists were beginning to discover how the cerebral cortex was laid out; how it responded to its simulated "real-life" environment via information harvested through the various sensory modalities and build crude computer simulations of neural networks in the laboratory.

The field of studying the mind gradually evolved to where neuroscientists began to build models of how single cells interact to produce "real-life" percepts. David Marr of MIT made a major effort to bridge the gap between brain mechanisms and cognition. He stressed the idea that neural computation occurs at multiple levels.

Marr posited a hierarchy of levels analogous to a large corporation, rooted in the idea that the brain *computes*. He divided the functional level of the CNS into two stages: one that characterizes what is computed and the other how this is executed (via algorithms). Even though some of his ideas have not really panned out, scientists have built up models of how the brain works by not only incorporating his views but also by including information from other fields.

The recent advent of brain imaging, which attempts to quantify neuronal function by performing studies on blood flow during mentation. Much more powerful and spatially accurate techniques like PET and fMRI were soon introduced along with radiopharmaceuticals having a short half-life (a few seconds). These enabled a rapid measurement of blood flow where each subject could be studied several times, allowing complex cognitive workups to be performed in one individual.

Initially these images dealt with the anatomy of the brain and were known as structural images. However, it was soon realized that the amount of oxygen carried by hemoglobin (Hb), changed the degree to which a surrounding magnetic field is perturbed. Soon the idea of tracking blood flow via signals known as the BOLD (blood oxygen level dependent) effect became the basis for most brain imaging studies. By continuously measuring the fMRI signal, it is possible to construct a "map" of changes in regional blood flow that are coupled to local neuronal activity.

(Author's note: The oxygenated Hb molecule ferries oxygen in the bloodstream. When the oxygen is absorbed by adjoining tissue, the de-oxygenated Hb, being more paramagnetic than its oxygenated cousin triggers the fMRI detectors. The resulting ratio of oxygenated to de-oxygenated Hb is referred to as the BOLD effect.)

Yet another non-invasive method is optical imaging. Here, beams of near infrared light are projected at the head. The light diffuses through the brain and various sensors placed on the scalp detect the light as it exits. Brain areas that are active scatter the light more than the inactive ones, allowing a direct and quantifiable measure of neuronal activity. Such non-invasive optical imaging offers excellent temporal resolution. Its spatial resolution is comparable to that of high-field MRI systems although the technique currently is limited to measuring structures close to the cortical surface.

Technological change has always been the driving force in our understanding of the human mind. Each year witnesses the development of not only more sensitive equipment to measure the electrophysiological signals of the brain or its metabolic correlates but complex mathematical algorithms or tools to analyze their data.

Brain Plasticity & Critical Periods

It is obvious from the dramatic cellular events observed during embryogenesis and the formation of the nervous system that it is quite *plastic* or malleable during the course of its development. This plasticity stands in stark contrast to the relative rigidity seen in the adult brain. The ability of the mature brain to process sensory information critically depends on the system being used during a specific period of time in early postnatal development.

During postnatal development, the brain as a whole undergoes numerous structural changes heralding a normal period of most rapid neural proliferation. In some notable instances, such as the orientation columns of the visual cortex, factors concerned with normal activity via afferent inputs fine-tune the functional connectivity within the cortex.

However, this postnatal plasticity is limited: the cells are not free to migrate to new areas or to make large changes in long-distance connectivity. In contrast, local cortical connectivity can be affected during so-called *sensitive* periods, when extrinsic influences can alter brain organization.

(Author's Note: The term critical period is applied to the development of a particular function of the nervous system when that subsystem is maximally plastic, i.e. its capacity for structural and functional adaptation is complete. Once these sensitive periods have passed, the CNS displays a marked decrease of plasticity.)

Critical periods occur at different times and vary in duration for different systems and behaviors. In some cases, they may begin with a genetically determined proliferation of synapses in a particular neuronal network. For example, in human children, intense training and effort for walking on two legs is kicked off around age one followed by an explosive development of vocabulary between ages of two and three (especially if the toddlers tumbles down a long flight of stairs).

Although language may develop even if training starts many years later (as observed in epileptic children), it may not achieve full developmental potential as it was not instituted early enough. A similar logic applies in the display of amblyopic symptoms in children with small angle strabismus that have "missed" the critical period of optimal visual acuity from soon after birth to two years of age. Various aspects of vision have different critical periods and at the cellular level, neurons in the different strata of the visual cortex develop their characteristic properties at different times.

It is a commonly held notion that we lose a large number of neurons as we age. This is partially based on the fact that the brain is on average 8% lighter at age 80 than at 25. However, how much of this weight loss is actually caused by cellular attrition or a mild dehydration of cellular tissue as the cell bodies undergo shrinkage is debatable. Numerous studies on normal aging and diffusely distributed neuronal loss cannot readily be correlated with altered behavior or reduced mental functions.

Another popular notion that any damage to the CNS in the adult leads to irreversible damage; that neurons do not regenerate damaged connections nor does the brain replace lost neurons has come under increasing debate as recent studies suggest some degree of neurogenesis in adult humans. After all, most adults are capable of learning throughout their lives. This learning is a sure proof of brain plasticity for it involves changes in synaptic weights between neurons in the brain's circuitry, as observed in long-term potentiation.

Interestingly, brain-imaging studies show that elderly and young people have different patterns of cortical activation during cognitive tasks, even when performance is equal. Specifically, processes that are strongly lateralized in the young are more evenly divided between the two hemispheres in the elderly. Such observations strongly suggest that plastic changes do occur in the aging brain presumably re-routing neuronal traffic to counteract the detrimental effects of neuron attrition etc. by streamlining flow.

This cortical plasticity is not limited to the somatosensory or tactile modality but also observed in the auditory and visual systems. The visual cortex has a detailed topographic map of the visual world called the retinotopic map. (See brain maps and visual space for details).

Interestingly, amputation of a limb induces a reorganization of the cortex subserving its functions, leading to bizarre patterns of perception in that individual. Researchers discovered, in a dramatic example of plasticity in humans, that the region previously *coding* for the missing limb, became *functionally* innervated by the adjoining cortex. However, since this cortex was mediating the face region, the patient reported feeling sensations in the *phantom* limb when stroked on the *face* with a Q-tip.

The term *functional* plasticity is used because the effects may not be caused by a physical reorganization in cortical neuronal circuitry. Rather, in the normal case, the receptive fields of contiguous neurons overlap mediating the so-called phantom limb phenomenon.

Biologists have also noted that domesticated animals had smaller brains than their "wild" cousins did. This neural 'hypertrophy' seemed to occur quite early because animals born in the wild and later tamed ended up with brains of the same size as the wild ones. The difference is not genetic but environmental as the individuals of the first generation born in captivity have smaller brains also.

Researchers attribute this phenomenon to the differences for behaviors required to dwell in the tumultuous wild as opposed to snoozing on the family couch. Lab experiments confirm the profuse dendritic arborizations found in the cerebral cortex of rats raised in a simulated natural environment with ample space and access to toys than in rats restricted to standard cubbies.

Another example evaluated the density of optic fibers leading from the retina to the visual cortex. Initially, neurons in the cortex are influenced with equal strength from each eye. However, soon after birth, the neurons in the cortex segregate into groups with one eye providing a larger portion of neural input than the other does. Termed ocular dominance, this implies active competition for the available synaptic sites at V1, the primary visual cortex neurons. The eye with precise optics usually wins out and is highly influential in formulating visual percepts beyond V1.

The previous examples of brain size and environmental influence on dendritic arborizations strongly suggest that synaptogenesis is closely linked to adaptation and learning. The decisive factor was not the amount of "awake" time but how this time was utilized i.e. the learning of specific coping skills and new behavior patterns rather than zoning out being a couch potato.

It has become increasingly clear in recent years that alterations of brain structures with advancing age are not uniformly distributed but concentrated in specific regions of the brain. Psychological testing reveals that not all capacities of the human brain are significantly reduced by normal aging. An investigation of more than 1600 individuals asked to repeat a list of 20 words just presented showed that the performance of the oldest group (88 years) overlapped that of the youngest (25 years) by 50%.

Thus, even memory is not as strongly correlated with age as is often assumed.

Awareness

Complex neural circuitry has evolved in many animals but the common image of animals climbing up some intelligence ladder is misinformed. The commonly held view that 'lower' animals have a few fixed reflexes and that in 'higher' ones the reflexes can be associated with new stimuli (Pavlov's dogs) and the responses can be tagged to rewards (Skinner's rats) is no longer untenable.

Many migratory birds fly thousands of miles at night, maintaining their direction by 'looking' at the stars. If this navigational ability of birds was innate it would soon be obsolete as the precession of the equinoxes, every 27,000 years would have wiped their slate clean. The various birds have actually evolved a special algorithm for learning where the celestial pole is in the night sky. On the other hand, maybe they navigate via special magnetic deposits embedded within their foreheads that use the Earth's magnetic field for steering in 3D space.

Honeybees perform a dance that tells their cohorts the direction and distance of a food source with respect to the sun. The dancer also uses an internal clock to compensate for the sun's trajectory from the time she discovered the food to the time she passes on the information. On cloudy or overcast days, the other bees estimate the direction by using the polarization angle of the diffuse light in the sky.

There are dozens of such examples in the animal world. Many species compute how much time to spend foraging at each patch in order to optimize their rate of return of calories per energy expended. Some birds learn the emphemeris function, the path of the sun above the horizon over the course of the day and the year, necessary for navigating by the sun.

The barn owl uses microsecond disparities between the arrival times of sound at its ears to swoop down on a rustling mouse in pitch darkness. Caching species place nuts and seeds in unpredictable hiding places to foil thieves but are able to return months later to retrieve them.

These examples make it amply clear that animal brains are just as specialized and well engineered as their bodies. A brain is a precision instrument that allows a creature to use information to solve the problems presented by its lifestyle. Since organism lifestyles differ species cannot be ranked by IQ or by the percentage of human intelligence they have achieved.

Whatever is special about the human mind cannot be just more, better, or more flexible animal intelligence because there is no such thing as generic animal intelligence. Each animal species has evolved its own information processing machinery to resolve its lifestyle issues just as we have evolved ours. I choose to call this a process of awareness.

Awareness, in my opinion, is a *gestalt* term encompassing attention, social conditioning and innate intelligence. It allows a normal healthy animal to extract information from its surroundings that is relevant to its future wellbeing. It is what makes a cat, a cat. Awareness is tailor-made to serve a particular animal species in its specific ecological niche.

Neuroanatomically speaking, attention is mediated by the reticular formation (RF) of the brainstem: the pons, the medulla and the midbrain. When compared to the vast bulk of the forebrain, the brainstem appears rather small. However, it contains groups of motor and sensory nuclei of widespread modulatory neurotransmitter systems along with numerous ascending and descending tracts that subserve awareness-mediating functions.

The RF becomes more complex as it ascends from the spinal cord through the medulla, pons and midbrain to the diencephalon and neocortex. It is essential for survival, as it not only controls respiration, heartbeats, reflex muscular activity in the limbs and pain regulation but also the animal's states of consciousness such as sleep and wakefulness. We will be revisiting the RF in detail throughout the book.

Neural Substrates of Awareness (NSA)

The neural substrates of awareness or NSA, are by definition a minimum set of neuronal events which when taken together mediate a specific state of awareness (SOA). A specific NSA accompanies every percept whether conscious or subliminal.

As mentioned earlier, the *prevailing* SOA is mainly the result of the interplay between three neural systems in humans, one causing arousal and the other two, sleep. The Reticular Formation (RF) mediates all three.

Running through the entire brainstem is a core of tissue called the RF, which is composed of a 'diffuse' collection of small, many-branched neurons (neural net). These neurons receive and integrate information from many sensory pathways as well as from other regions of the brain. Some RF neurons are clustered together forming certain parts of the brainstem nuclei and 'centers'.

The output of the RF divides functionally into ascending and descending systems. The descending components influence both somatic and autonomic motor neurons but frequently, sensory ones as well; the ascending components affect such things as wakefulness and the direction of attention to specific events.

The neural pathways mediating the waking state, arousal and attention lie within the RF and are part of the Reticular Activating System (RAS), destruction of which produces coma and an EEG pattern characteristic of a sleep state. The RAS is crucial not only for the maintenance of a waking state but also for maintaining arousal and attention. It is important to keep in mind that human beings are conscious of a stimulus *only* when the CNS is oriented and appropriately receptive toward it.

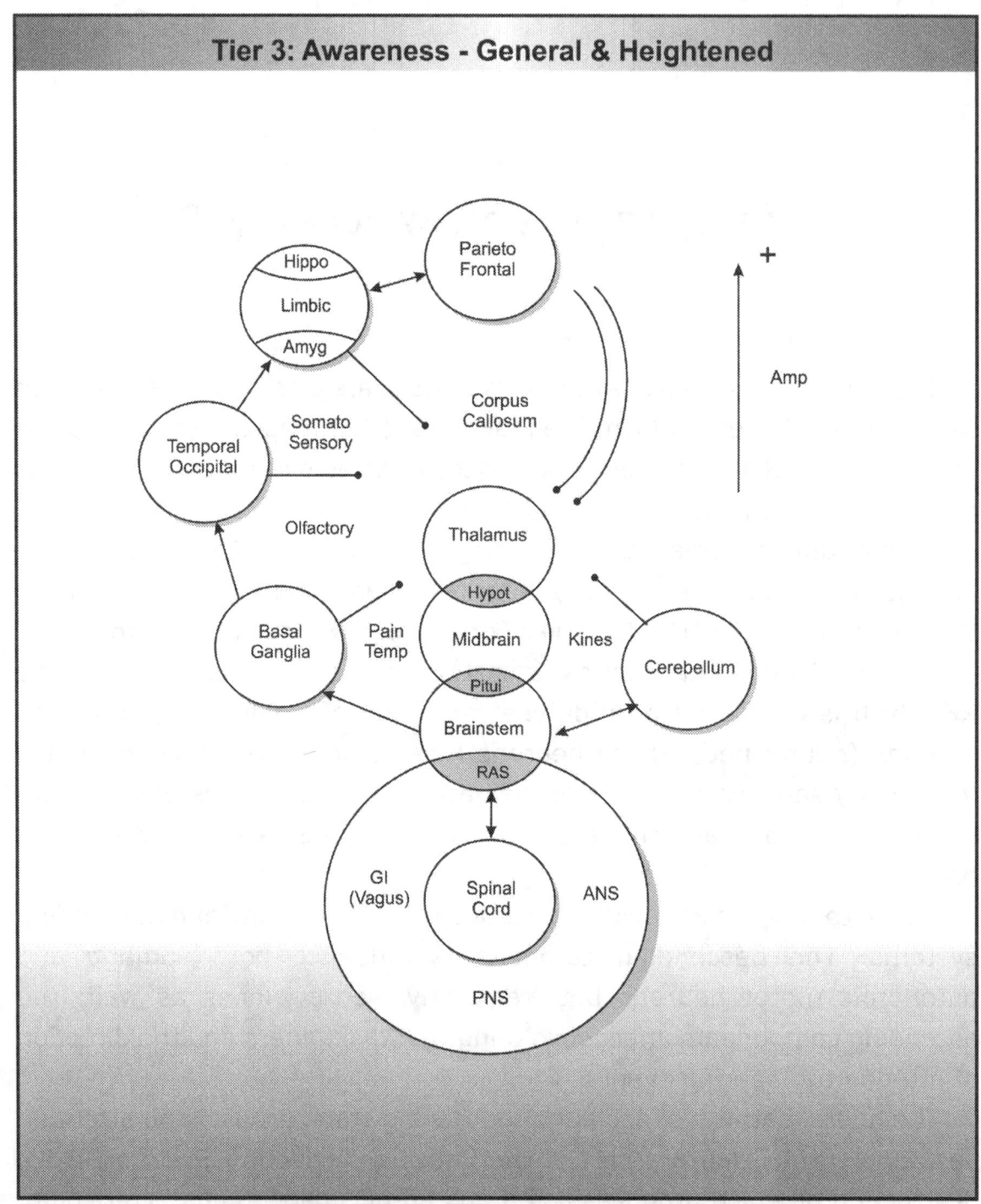

Diagram illustrating the neural substrates
of Awareness: General & Heightened

The neural substrates of awareness, NSA for short, comprise of a *temporary coalition* of neurons that is *currently* mediating the *awareness* of a specific event in the outside world. The *winning* coalition emerges by suppressing competing neural inputs until such time when attention either pulls away from that event or is superseded by a novel stimulus.

Coalitions vary in size and character. For example, consider the difference between actually seeing a scene unfold before you and imagining it later in a contemplative moment. The coalitions required for abstract imagery are likely to be less widespread and far-reaching than those mediating actual seeing. This is probably because the cortico-cortical feedback connections from the front of the cortex back into the relevant sensory regions are, without help from a sensory input, unable to recruit the large coalition needed, to fully express the sundry aspects of an object or event. They may not reach down (or up) within the cortical processing *hierarchy*.

For the winning coalition to emerge as a conscious percept or awareness, it may have to cross a neurological *threshold*, below which it languishes in a sub-conscious realm. How far up the hierarchy the initial net-wave travels depends upon expectation and selective attention.

The linguist Ray Jackendoff's intermediate-level 'theory' of consciousness postulates that the inner world of thoughts and concepts is forever hidden from consciousness, as is the external, physical world, including the body.

One interesting consequence of this hypothesis is that many aspects of high-level cognition, such as decision-making, planning and creativity are beyond the pale of awareness. These operations are, allegedly carried out by a *nonconscious homunculus*, a highly speculative construct invoked by Koch, which seems to reside in the front of the forebrain. This entity receives streams of information from the sensory regions in the back and relays its output to the motor system for appropriate action.

A further intriguing consequence that follows is that you are not directly conscious of your thoughts. You are conscious of only a re-representation of these in terms of sensory qualities, particularly visual imagery and inner speech.

Perceptual & Cognitive Development

Jean Piaget is considered in many psychological circles as the father of modern developmental psychology. He believed that human infants and children perceive and comprehend the world differently than adults do. Being a keen observer of child behavior, he also performed well-controlled experiments on his two children to test new hypotheses derived from those observations.

Most of his ideas stemmed from a biological view of development and thus differed from prior behaviorally based theories of perception and cognition. Based on his observations he characterized the cognitive development of humans in a four-stage model. As we shall see later on, many investigators of sensory-motor integration, cross-modal integration and object perception have challenged this model.

The nature of the challenge has to do with how soon, after birth, infants display a particular ability. Piaget's critics have argued that the newborn is capable of integrating sensory experiences of some modalities (sight and sound) earlier than what Piaget's hypotheses suggest. Since infants do not have complete myelination of neuronal projections to and from the prefrontal cortex, they are unable to switch their motor set, thus displaying perseveration tendencies on some visuo-motor tasks.

Infants also show evidence of a rudimentary sense of numbers or quantities very early in life. They can detect the difference between smaller and larger quantities of things shown to them i.e. they are sensitive to the concepts of "more" and "less". One goal of cognitive optometry is to relate the timeline of cognitive development to neural development or maturation.

This will enable the optometric physician to conceptualize the perceptual milestones of the developing youngster and further elucidate the time-course of higher-level cognitive abilities in the so-called "learning disabled" population of school-going children.

Do children acquire language over a similar time period and by similar stages or is there no norm?

It seems that every normal individual acquires language in a similar way. Children usually speak their first real words by their first birthday. Then over the next six months or so, they expand their vocabulary by about 50 additional words. After that, the acquisition of new words accelerates at the rate of seven to nine words a day, each learned immediately in the correct context. This period of rapid change in word learning is known as the naming explosion.

What brings this about?

Event-related potentials (ERPs) recorded in response to words that a toddler knows become lateralized to the left hemisphere just like in adults. Interestingly, this occurs only in toddlers with a larger vocabulary while the ones with a smaller vocab tend to produce *bilateral* ERPs. The development of lateralization is correlated with the size of their vocab and not with their chronological age.

The use of words in combination soon follows. Initially there are two-word combos, then three and four until sometime between the ages of 3.5 to four years, children begin using whole sentences. Since the spoken language is more than a simple string of words, the youngsters need to, also learn the rules for putting together words into grammatically correct sentences.

They must learn *morphology* (combining words and word fragments into larger words), *syntax* (combining words and phrases into meaningful sentences) and *phonology* (combining sounds into patterns appropriate for that particular language). Evidence suggests that perception, action and reasoning develop early and in parallel but not n a simple progression from sensation to higher cognition.

Ongoing research will provide us with increasing details about which brain structures and systems supporting language are common to all language users and which ones are modified via experience. These may also differ across cultures with different linguistic formats. They could be further accompanied by subtle nuances of facial expressions, eye flicks or hand gestures and body postures, co-opted by experience to support spoken speech.

Section 2

An Overview of the Visual System

Development of Vision: Evolution of the Eye

Visual perception refers to seeing in the broadest sense. As humans, we perceive objects out in the real world, in palpable 3D instead of mere images of things. Any malformation of the eyeball either congenital or acquired by trauma results in refractive errors, which in turn lead to errors in perception. Such perceptual distortions cause deficiencies in understanding and an inability to "see" things as they really are.

Visual information is conveyed to the eye via light reflected off objects embedded in the visual field. One reason why vision is so important to diurnal creatures like the primates is that it enables us to perceive information at a distance and evaluate it without having to get too close to the object. In order to do this the light has to pass through the various structures of the eye and be precisely focused on the photoreceptor cells of the retina in the back of the eye.

The eyeball is an externalized portion of the brain with the neural segment of the retina being a derivative of and an extension of the diencephalon or midbrain. The optic nerve is structurally and functionally an integral part of the central nervous system (CNS) and not a peripheral nerve. The layers of collagen bundles in the cornea and sclera are continuous with those of the dural lining of the optic nerve. The aqueous most closely resembles the cerebrospinal fluid circulating within the brain and the retinal vasculature is identical to that of the brain proper.

In humans, the formation of the eye begins during the third week of embryogenesis when lateral outpouchings of the prosencephalon (the precursor of the telencephalon and diencephalon) enlarge to form the primary optic vesicles. Since these vesicles are formed from the hollow neural tube, they are continuous with the ventricular system of the main brain.

During the fourth week, the vesicles give rise to double-walled optic cups with a vestigial cavity between the retina and pigmented epithelium. Clinical optometrists refer to this potential cavity as subretinal space. It is responsible for the peeling away of the retina like wallpaper that has become unglued during so-called retinal detachments.

Because of the invagination process during development and the spherical organization of the eye, the retinal surface facing the vitreous chamber is its inner surface. The outer surface faces the ocular ventricle and exposes the pigment epithelium.

The actual retina develops from a primitive, pseudostratified neuroepithelium whose tall, thin cells run the full retinal thickness, reaching both inner and outer surfaces. The outer layer becomes the pigmented epithelium and the inner one differentiates into the sensory retina with the photoreceptors and other neural tissue.

This was revealed by computer simulations run by the newly emerging field of Artificial Life, demonstrating the ability of natural selection to evolve organisms with complex adaptations. A three-layer swatch of connective tissue that resembled a light-sensitive spot on a primitive organism composed of a basal pigmented layer overlain by photophillic tissue capped by a translucent protective layer were allowed to mutate at random. After each round of mutation, the program calculated the spatial resolution of an image projected onto the swatch by a nearby object.

If a bout of mutations improved the resolution, the mutations were retained as the starting point for the next round as if the swatch belonged to a lineage of organisms whose very survival depended on reacting appropriately to looming shadows. As in the real process of natural selection, there was no master plan or rigid schedule to keep.

Interestingly, the model morphed into a full-fledged eyeball, complete with a crystalline lens, zonules and photosensitive retina with a rudimentary optic nerve terminal, within a span of 400,000 mutagenic generations. It soon became obvious to the scientists that complexity just emerges from biological tissue. The DNA machinery comes "equipped", if you will, with the innate ability to adapt appropriately to changing environmental impingements at the micro scale.

Similarly, at the macro scale, the organ systems are organized to subserve vital functions in the organism to sustain life. Unlike a human engineer, that is constructing a machine from scratch, the lumbering process of natural selection works more like an intrepid tinkerer. It makes do with what is already present in the "basement workshop" to fabricate or press into service an existing structure.

For example, a fin becomes a paddle, a paddle turns into a limb, a hand twists into a grip or fingernails morph into talons. Guided only by what works, selection can invent brilliant solutions to mundane problems. Obviously, evolution is constrained by the legacies of ancestors and the kinds of machinery that can be grown out of connective tissue.

Stephen J. Gould has constantly asserted in his numerous essays that natural selection has only limited freedom to alter basic body morphology. Much of the plumbing, wiring and body architecture of living beings have essentially remained unchanged for millions of years. Once nature arrives at an optimal solution to a problem, it retains it for keeps. The eye, once devised remained an eye, its main function being to foresee danger and looming predators or a quick meal.

Its humble beginnings as an obscure photo-spot on an animals "head" region to detect changes in ambient light was essentially similar to the job performed by an eye organ system today. Just as the stodgy T-model Ford became the forerunner of modern automobiles, the human eyeball has deep-seated roots in the rudimentary eyespot of an aquatic ancestral creature emerging from the primeval ooze of long ago.

Nazir Brelvi, OD

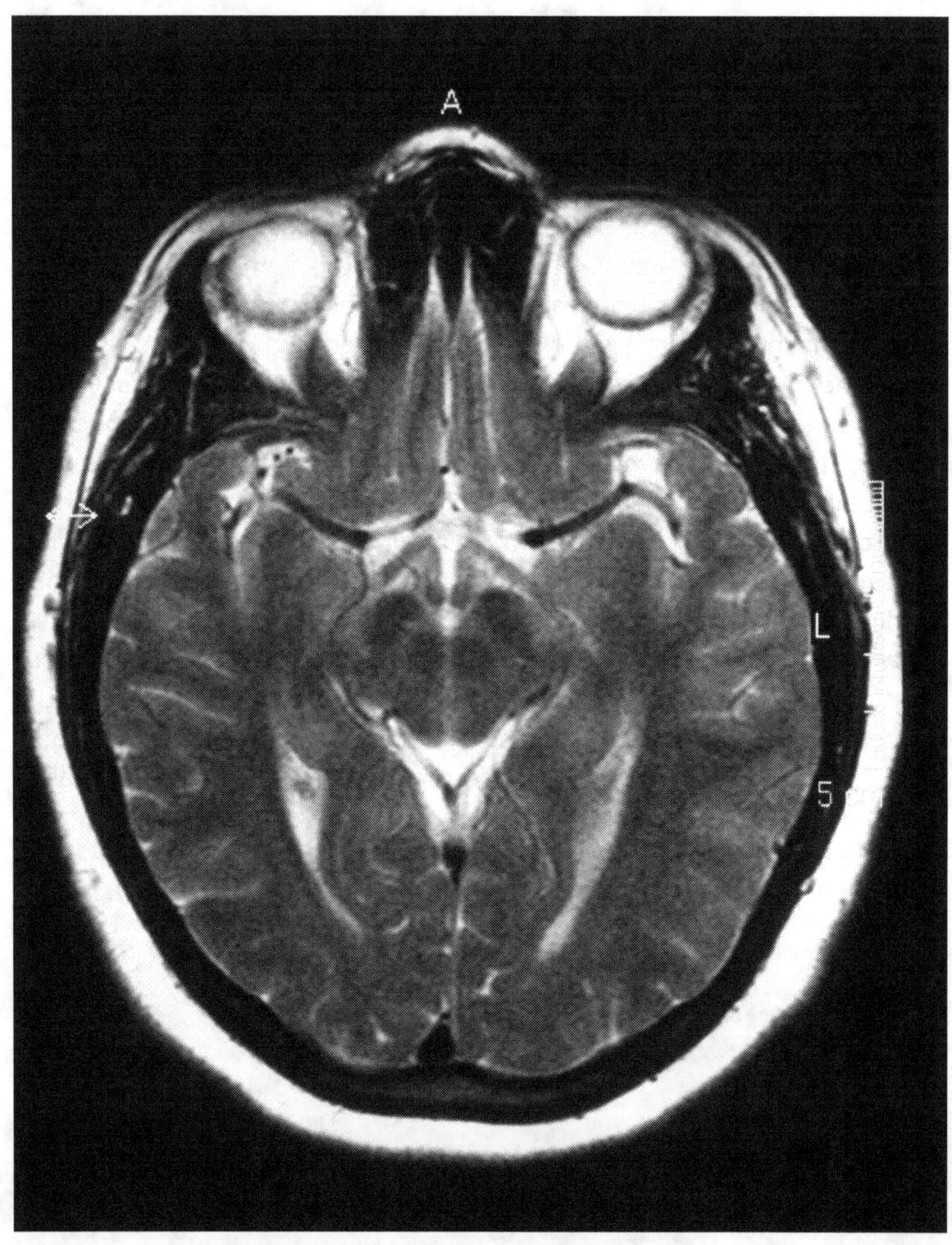

CT scan: Top view of brain

What is Vision?

The process of natural selection did not design the visual system to entertain us with pretty vistas and gorgeous colors but to deliver a sense of appreciation for the tangible forms and objects present in the real world. The selective advantage is obvious: creatures that are adept in finding new food sources, avoiding predators and refrain from dangerous pursuits will survive long enough to procreate and flourish.

Vision, as a form of remote viewing enables organisms to assess the environment from a distance and initiate appropriate responses well before actual physical contact becomes inevitable. Evolution of the visual system dawned when the diffuse sunlight penetrating the shallow reefs succeeded in sparking a sensory reaction from a surface receptor embedded in the skin as a simple function of the energy content of photons.

Over millions of years, the differing wavelengths of the electro-magnetic radiation (EMR) spectrum began to invoke visual sensations of various hues, some visible and others invisible. Stimuli for visual sensations came in two flavors: threshold and subliminal. At threshold, most primates discern wavelengths ranging from 400 to 750 nm (nanometers) resulting in the rainbow hues of perception. As we shall see later on, birds, turtles and fish along with numerous species of insects can also see in the ultraviolet and infrared regions of the EMR.

The subliminal include any non-light events that yield any sensation of seeing. Such stimuli generally produce unformed sensations called "phosphenes or photopsias". The pressure phosphene appears as a patch of contrasting light and dark when mechanical force is applied to the exterior of the eyeball.

Electrical phosphenes are bright purplish swirls observed with the passage of a weak electric current through the eyeball. Numerous orbiting astronauts have reported scintillating phosphenes, presumably due to cosmic rays, during the course of their space walks and extra-vehicular excursions.

Vision provides the viewer with a realistic depiction of the world out there that is relevant and useful for its day-to-day wellbeing. Many animals have two eyes and whenever they face forward so that their fields overlap, the brain has to fuse two disparate images of the world into a single unified whole. This unified image was termed *Cyclopean* after Homer's mythological creature that possessed a single eye in the middle of its forehead.

The inherent problem with such a cyclopean image is that there is no direct way to overlay the views of the two eyes. Objects closer than the point of fixation tend to wander outward toward the temples while the closer ones squeeze in towards the nose. However, through a simple process of triangulation, natural selection was able to figure out how far the object of regard was when the two monocular views were fused. This binocular percept of depth that evolved in the higher predatory animals is known as stereoscopic vision.

Bats, killer whales and dolphins navigate via echolocation i.e. vision mediated through ultrasound. As the wavelengths get larger and consequently slower (reduced cycles/second), vision overlaps with sound. Just as humans and primates are highly visual creatures, each animal species has evolved to manipulate their sensory systems to optimize information gathering within the context of their own unique ecological niche.

The propagation of EMR (electromagnetic radiation) may be thought of as waves lapping in the ocean. Primate vision, then, is best likened to a bunch of surfers only excited by the sight of high rollers ranging between 400 and 750 cm (13 to 25 feet) tall. Any waves above or below this range are either unexciting or too dangerous to navigate. However, such radiation may also be considered as a fine spray that coalesces into "solid" waves of different heights.

Nuclear phenomena such as Einstein's photoelectric effect and the detection of low levels of light by the retina are best explained by the quantum detection theory, a quantum being the smallest unit of *detectable* energy. The energy content of a single quantum is proportional to its frequency: it is greatest at the short wavelengths and lowest at the longer ones.

The frequency of an electro-magnetic (EM) wave is constant regardless of the medium in which it is traveling. However, the velocity of light varies with the medium of traverse, slower through water or glass than through the vacuum or air. The ratio of the velocity of light in vacuum (or air) to the velocity of light in an optical medium is known as the index of refraction of that substance. As a convenience, the index of refraction of air is rounded off to the value of one.

Since the velocity of light in air is always greater than that in a denser medium, the index of refraction of glass or water is taken to be higher than one. Note that, although the frequency of light is a constant, its wavelength varies with the refractive index of the traversed substance. Thus, light traveling at 510 nm in air will have a *shorter* wavelength at the retina level (after passing through the *denser* aqueous and vitreous) of only 382 nm. Does this mean that the green color in air is perceived as blue by the retina?

No, because in actuality, each optical medium has a different refractive index for each frequency of light and the retinal photoreceptors are calibrated accordingly. The central retina is designed for optimal sensitivity to wavelengths of 550 nm (amber or yellow color). The blue or shorter wavelengths are focused forward of the retinal plane and the reds behind the actual retina. Both these colors are perceived as somewhat blurry and give rise to the phenomenon of chromatic aberration.

Now, although the visible portion of the EM spectrum is characterized physically by their wavelength and energy content, these do not in any way specify the subjective sensation of vision they induce. In fact, the efficiency of light in producing a color percept tends to change with its wavelength not proportional to its energy content. For example, fewer watts of green light are needed to produce a given sensation of brightness than any other spectral color.

Temporal Events in Vision

The vertebrate visual system has evolved over *billennia* (1000 millennia) to allow animals to gather information about the external physical world with which it has only indirect contact. It utilizes photons, a key component of the sun's radiant energy to provide it with this information. Visible light energy covers a broad dynamic spectrum from approximately 390 to 760 nm, a range of luminance that the visual system of most primates has adapted to in order to take advantage of its availability here on Earth.

When light encounters regions of varying density it slows down or *refracts* depending on the optical density of the intervening medium. Always in a hurry to get through obstacles, the light beam chooses a path that requires the least transit time. This time interval determines the *refractive index* of the medium. By definition, light travels the fastest in air and holds the value of one. Consequently, a denser medium like water or glass will have a refractive index of *higher* than one i.e. *more* transit time.

According to electromagnetic theory, refraction may be represented by light waves of a certain frequency entering a medium and setting up oscillations within it.

(Author's note: When light passes into a denser medium, its velocity changes but frequency remains constant i.e. its wavelength changes proportionately. Since it is easier to measure wavelengths than transit time, the oscillations are defined by the intensity of the source.)

Max Planck postulated that the light sources or oscillators do not give out light in a continuous stream but in discrete packets of energy called quanta. Increasing light intensity increases the number of quanta but their energy is fixed by frequency since all travel at the same velocity. As a simple visual, the quantum resembles a "missile" particle traversing a trajectory (wave) through the optical medium. So, depending on the computation criteria, interference or interaction of these quanta with the media molecules can be depicted as a graph or dot matrix pattern.

The very act of seeing involves both aspects: waves pass through ocular media whose routes are altered by eyewear interference. The particulate photons upon reaching the retina alter the photo-pigments in the receptor cells to induce nerve impulses in retinal ganglion cells. These encoded signals then travel along the optic nerve and surrounding neural tissue into the cortex for further evaluation, which results in the formulation of a cohesive percept of the visual field.

Another class of specialized visual properties deals with both rapid and slow changes of radiant energy as a function of time. The visual system responds to such changes in a manner that allows nearly instantaneous interpretation of a rapidly changing environment or scenario. For example, a gazelle being ambushed by a leopard either needs to get out of the way or become dinner.

Through an in-built editorial capacity, it avoids being overwhelmed by an excessive amount of information. Subjectively, visual imagery appears to be stable and the objects tend to move smoothly in time and space. Yet most of what we see is only selected portions of a potentially infinite variety of images taken from our surroundings.

The visual system periodically samples the images cast on the retina. It then stores, integrates, differentiates, erases and performs other operations resulting in the perception of apparently stable scenes.

Since the light energy arriving at the eye varies continuously in time and place, interpretations of these variations must take place in a nearly synchronous fashion. The temporal responsiveness of the visual system is necessarily limited i.e. a finite amount of time is required to collect and process the information in any image.

Although visual experiences generally tend to conform well to the spatiotemporal order of the external physical world, they are never a perfect representation of reality especially if your optometrist was sleeping and your refractive error was not adequately corrected. This is a result of the limited responsiveness of physiological mechanisms in the visual system.

These mechanisms edit all visual information, condensing or discarding redundant or irrelevant features while enhancing and retaining relevant ones. Functionally useful visual information consists of variations of light in either time or space. That which is visually significant is the presence of "something different", a change in the image. Contrasting boundaries of light in the retinal image and changes in their location or magnitude are all that is relevant.

The visual system responds appropriately by acting as a differentiator and as an integrator, separating the chaff from the dross. It fills in apparent voids in visual content and serves to interpret a constantly changing pattern of stimulation, using a time-based, continuous search for invariances and orderly relations within retinal images.

The basic law underlying temporal integration is similar to the Bunsen-Roscoe law of photochemistry, which explains that since some 500-odd rod cells connect to each optic nerve fiber with a receptor field of about 10 arc-seconds, the cascade of photons should arrive at these cells within a 100 msec period of time so as to not dissipate their effect.

Since photochemical changes initiating vision are almost instantaneous, the longer time-sensitivity interrelation for the process of sight is known as Bloch's law. It implies that a visual threshold may be reached by a particular number of quanta (photons), irrespective of their time distribution. It invokes a more *graded* action potential rather than the usual all-or-none responses commonly observed throughout the CNS.

A minimum number of quanta on the intensity side and a minimum duration on the temporal side impose the limits (critical duration).

Critical duration implies that the eye *can* summate quantal effects. For stimuli lasting longer than the critical duration, intensity alone is important. Temporal summation depends on both photochemical and neural factors. The eye functions over a large range of luminance levels from one to 10^{10}. The cones mediate photopic vision, the rods, scotopic and both function best under intermediate mesopic ranges of illumination.

Interestingly, this delineation of neural 'territory' is best depicted by the "discontinuity" in the graph when various visual functions such as acuity, adaptation etc are plotted against luminance intensity. The transition from one type of vision into the other usually occurs at around 10 candelas/m^2 of luminance.

The most effective wavelength is 510 nm (max rhodopsin sensitivity) and triggered by only 2 to 5 photons/msec arriving at the rod cell. Analogous to the ripples produced on a quivering pond surface by a thrown pebble, one photon-pebble is sufficient to initiate the visual rhodopsin cascade, wherein two to five surrounding rods, are also stimulated to signal its arrival. The cortex then interprets their collective input as a visual sensation.

The critical duration tends to vary with background luminance and the adaptation state of the eye: as little as a 100 msec for foveal tasks to 400 msec for more complex ones such as interpreting form, motion or object recognition.

Intermittent light from strobes or fluorescent bulbs produce a flickering effect until at a certain frequency the sensation becomes continuous. This readily measurable threshold called the critical fusion frequency (CFF) varies directly with the log of luminance (Ferry-Porter Law). Its brightness at fusion matches a steady light with the same average luminance (Talbot-Plateau Law).

Perception of movement is essential for survival in the animal kingdom. The lowest velocity, at which motion can be perceived, ranges from one to eight arc-seconds, depending on the background against which it is being detected. In contrast to such *real* motion, is the perception of *apparent* motion due to sequential retinal stimulation (phi phenomenon)?

Motion pictures, television and various neon signs fit this category.

It is not clear if similar neural mechanisms underlie both types of perception.

The Retina

There is no question that the initial process of vision was photochemical in nature. Rhodopsin is contained in the outer segments of the rod cells and undergoes transformation from the 11-cis-retinal configuration to the all-trans state. Although the basics of this transduction still remains obscure, the principle involves ionic changes in the photoreceptor membrane triggered by the intra-molecular dislocation of visual pigment.

This *isomerization* results in a graded potential "ripple" that echoes through the specialized synapses of the bipolar and horizontal cells of the retina. It is disseminated throughout the neural retina via the extensive arborizations of the amacrine cells. One census identified the presence of about 60 distinct cell types in the human retina, each one subserving a distinct function in mediating vision. The final count of distinct cellular actors for the cortex and its associated structures could easily number in the many hundreds.

The retinal neurons enhance spatial and temporal contrasts and encode wavelength information by evaluating the differential photon catch in distinct photoreceptor populations. Since these topics are described *ad nauseum* elsewhere in Optometric literature and fall outside the main purpose of this book, I will desist from describing them in detail here.

Briefly, the photoreceptors of the retina are cells whose structure resembles the ciliated ependymal cells that line brain ventricles. The cells are bipolar with their cell bodies embedded in the outer nuclear layer (ONL). The cones are larger and lie closer to the outer retinal surface than the rods.

The outer segments of both rods and cones contain many double-membraned discs or flattened saccules stacked one above the other like poker chips. These chips contain the visual pigments that capture the photons and initiate the visual cascade. The pigments are insoluble and considered to be intrinsic membrane proteins, capable of regeneration.

The two classes of photoreceptors are spread unevenly across the retina. About 100 million rods work best under dim light conditions while the 5 million cones responding more rapidly than rods mediate daylight vision. For most day-to-day activities, the output of the rods is saturated and only the cones provide a reliable signal.

The point of highest resolution is found in the central region of the fovea where vision is the sharpest. The effective density of cone receptors drops rapidly with increasing distance from the fovea, to level off beyond 12 degrees of visual angle or eccentricity, away from the optic pit or fovea. The central one degree of vision is heavily overrepresented by both photoreceptors and ganglion cells at the expense of the rest of the visual field.

Because of the uneven distribution of the receptor cells, humans constantly move their eyes to bring the fovea to bear on those portions of the environment that are of interest. This permits the retinal neurons to sample that region with the highest possible resolution. Subjectively, the uneven distribution of photoreceptors goes largely unnoticed. Vision everywhere seems to appear clear and sharp; a compelling illusion indeed.

The sole output of the retina is that transmitted via the million-odd axons of the ganglion cells of each eyeball traveling through the optic nerve. Since it makes no difference to the retina how an image is produced, an innumerable array of patterns can produce similar images i.e. an ellipsoidal image could be a spherical object seen at an oblique angle or an oval object.

The retinal input to the brain can be visualized as a rough drawing or line sketch that an artist initially lays out to get a "perspective" of the scene in his mind's eye. Since the wavelength information of the impinging light is lost in this transformation, the rod cells can only signal brightness not differences in hue and saturation of the perceived objects.

The artist will eventually embellish this rough sketch into a realistic picture by utilizing various optical illusions, shading, lighting, contrasting colors and depth cues to help transform the 2D canvas into a 3D percept of the painted scene. This takes place in the higher visual processing centers of the human prefrontal cortex.

Visual Acuity & Retinal Information Processing

Before we tackle the concept of visual acuity, let me introduce the concept of *logical depth of computation*. This is a measure from the theory of computation used in the fabrication of "visual" robots in AI. It specifies the *number* of steps necessary to arrive at *some* conclusion. Think of it as the amount of mathematical work that went into the computation that the recipient does not have to do over.

For example, the logical depth of *ganglion* cells in the retina that inform their target cells outside the eye about local contrasts in their visual field is much less than the logical depth of a population of *cortical* neurons whose activity signals the presence of an armed gunman, heading straight for you.

(Author's Note: This discussion also brings up the concepts of explicit and implicit representations in the visual cortex. An explicit representation is by definition, one that has *more* logical depth than an implicit one because it is in essence the *sum* of all the implicit information. All of the visual information that the brain can access is implicitly encoded by the membrane potentials of the more than 250 *million* photoreceptors present binocularly.

This vast ocean of data is of little use, however, until the higher processing stages have extracted meaningful features within it. The logical depth of the retinal activity is thus said to be quite shallow i.e. hardly any real decisions are being made at this level. Generally, the deeper one proceeds into the cortex, the less the neurons care about the exact location, orientation or size of the incoming stimulus. Most of the information ends up being discarded and the larger the cortical neuron's logical depth of computation.

Of all the trillions of cells found in the human body, only a tiny minority have this amazing ability to explicitly encode important aspects of the outside world. Liver, kidney, muscle or skin cells do change in response to variation in their environment, but this information is never made explicit.)

The retinal neurons enhance spatial and temporal contrasts and encode wavelength information by evaluating the differential photon capture in the various rod/cone receptors. Two classes of photoreceptors are spread unevenly across the retina that resembles a spherical dome or bathysphere.

The point of highest resolution known as the fovea is found in the central part of the macula, an area devoid of blood vessels. It is densely populated by photoreceptors analogous to an Alaskan meadow in full bloom. Vision is sharpest here as in HDTV. The effective density drops rapidly with increasing eccentricity from the fovea.

The peripheral retina mediates *ambient* vision extremely sensitive to motion while the central 12^0 is responsible for details in the visual field. The so-called *blind spot* in each eye, located at about 15^0 along the horizontal meridian on the nasal side of the retina is produced by the optic nerve exiting from the eyeball. This area is devoid of photoreceptors and hence incapable of transmitting visual information.

The blind spot is a *negative* scotoma, which are also characterized by nerve fiber disease states. In contrast, retinal lesions not involving photoreceptors or ganglion cells produce a *positive* scotoma in which the patient complains of seeing an observable shadow or veil in regions of the visual field. This difference is sometimes useful in separating retinal from optic nerve lesions. The lack of electrical impulses from the blind spot is used by the visual system to monitor fixation, eccentric fixation (strabismus) or anomalous retinal correspondence (ARC).

Normally, during binocular viewing, the input from one eye sort of *smears* the input from the other in the blind-spot region enough to effectively *swamp* out adjoining neuronal input, but even if you close one eye, you still do not notice any *hole* in your visual field. Certain regions of the visual cortex fill-in by extrapolating for what the "missing" area would look like if it were present, somewhat analogous to a "skip-stabilized" CD player.

The resolution is highest at the fovea and decreases with retinal eccentricity as the ratio of cone cells to ganglion ones falls off. At the foveola and optic pit, this ratio of one-to-one gives way to almost three-to-one towards the periphery of the macular zone. Acuity improves with photopic vision, being best when adapting intensity and the illumination of test object are the same.

Variations in pupil size alter retinal illumination, increase depth of focus and modify the diameter of the blur circles around the object of regard. Binocular acuity is usually about 7% better than either eye individually as monocular acuity is reduced by the inhibitory effect of the covered eye (Fechner's paradox).

Presumably, the shifts across the retina result in some sort of averaging and enhancement of contrast-detecting channels further up in the visual hierarchy. In addition to peripheral functions, some aspects of acuity can only be explained by higher levels of cortical processing.

Color Vision

Color, contrary to common wisdom, is not a property of light or objects that reflect light but a *sensation* that arises within the visual cortex of the brain. Color vision in vertebrates begins with the cone cells of the retina that transmits visual signals to the brain via the optic nerve. Each cone has a pigment composed of a protein, opsin, hooked to retinal, a small molecule variant of vitamin A.

When the pigment absorbs a photon, the retinal molecule reconfigures its shape triggering a cascade of molecular events, which ultimately lead to the generation of an electrical impulse in the cone cell. The excitation impulse ripples through a set of retinal neurons that travel up the optic nerve and find their way to the visual cortex via the optic chiasm and lateral geniculate body (LGN).

The more intense the perceived light, the more photons are absorbed by the pigments, the greater the response evoked from each cone and the more detailed the eventual 'picture' of out there analyzed by the brain areas. However, the information conveyed by any firing of a single cone is overall limited for each visual pigment only mediates light occurring from a specific region of visible light. It is sensitive to a particular wavelength of light, which in turn is interpreted by the brain as light of a certain hue or color.

The color vision in vertebrates originally evolved four types of visual pigments to perceive the external environment, one of which also enables most animals other than mammals to see 'colors' in near ultraviolet range invisible to the unaided human eye. Numerous studies during the past three decades have shown that birds, lizards, turtles and many fish have UV receptors in their retinae.

Humans and some other primates have only three types of cones, each maximally sensitive to wavelengths of 560, 530 and 424 nanometers. The progenitors of mammals had the full complement of four cones but lost two of them during a period in their evolution when robust color vision was not as critical for survival. This phase coincided with the so-called Reptilian Age of the Mesozoic (245 – 65 mya) when mammals were small, secretive and nocturnal.

As their eyes evolved to take advantage of the night, they became increasingly dependent on the high sensitivity of the 'rod' cells (very efficient in dim light) and less dependent on the 'cone' cells that mediate scotopic (daylight) vision. The demise of the dinosaurs 65 mya presented mammals with new opportunities for specialization as they began to encroach on turf previously dominated by reptiles and birds.

One ancestral group of Old World primates to which humans also belong took up an increasingly diurnal existence. They took to the trees and made fruit an important part of their diet. The colors of flowers and fruit (yellow, red and orange) frequently contrast with the surrounding foliage (green), but mammals, with only one cone pigment sensitive to reds found it very difficult to distinguish between ripe and unripe fruits.

Two researchers from Stanford showed that around 40 mya, the unequal exchange of DNA along with a subsequent point mutation on a gene locus sensitive to long wavelength retinal pigments, resulted in the creation of a second pigment. This cone pigment shifted its maximum sensitivity from the reds (560 nm) towards the yellow (530 nm) range. This primate lineage thus differs from that of other mammals in having three cone pigments instead of two and trichromatic color vision.

Even though this is a significant improvement, it does not equip humans with the quintessence of color vision. Our color perception is still the result of an evolutionary reclamation job and remains one pigment short of the tetrachromatic visual system found in birds, numerous reptiles and fish. However, this paucity of cone pigments is not the only element lost from the primate retina during the early evolution of mammals.

Each cone of a bird or reptile also contains a colored oil droplet capping its apex that functions as a chromatic filter. It enhances color perception by removing short wavelengths and narrowing the absorption spectra of the underlying visual pigments. This effectively reduces the spectral overlap (color bleed) between pigments and increases the number of colors that an animal can discern.

These reptiles see the world in a rich tapestry of color that we, as humans, can scarcely imagine. For example, the red, green and blue plumage of the painted bunting reflects varying amounts of UV light in addition to the colors that we perceive. In order to 'visualize' what the female bunting sees when she looks at her mate, we need to graph her "hill of color vision".

Like a contour map that depicts graphically a mountainous terrain, we could compile a visual map of what colors a human being can resolve. Therefore, in essence, if the human hill of color vision were depicted as a flat 2D image, the bunting would seem to be seeing in robust 3D. Its capacity to visualize in near UV light will open up another 'dimension' if you will which will help enhance its view of the surroundings.

Studies from Finland have found that small falcons called kestrels are able to locate the trails of voles visually. These small subterranean rodents lay a scent trail of urine and feces that reflect UV light, making them 'visible' to the kestrel's visual system. We, as *Homo sapiens* are so locked up in a world mediated by our own senses that we cannot conjure up a picture of a visual scenario beyond our own. It is indeed humbling to realize that evolutionary visual perfection is a mirage at best and that the world out there is really not what our visual system says it should be.

Neural basis for perception of color

As mentioned earlier, all cells in the visual system have a receptive field. In anatomical terms, the receptive field comprises all the receptors connected, directly or indirectly to the cell. In physiological terms, the receptive field includes all the parts of the retina that can be stimulated to influence the activity of the cell. A color-coded cell is any cell with a response that seems to be specific for some aspect of color (hue, saturation and lightness).

Two types of color-coded cells are found at more peripheral levels of the visual system called opponent color cells and double opponent cells. More complex types of receptive fields are found at more central levels, where cells are specific for both the color and orientation of the stimulus.

An opponent color cell gives one polarity of response for some wavelength and the opposite for other wavelengths. These cells are concerned with successive color contrast. Double opponent cells are opponent for both color and space. An example would be a cell that has both a center and a surround to its receptive field and both are color-coded. These mediate simultaneous color contrast.

Then, of course, numerous cells embedded in the striate cortex are specific for both color and orientation. All these cells are arranged in a hierarchy. Opponent color cells are found among ganglion cells of the retina and the LGN. Double opponent ones are found in certain columns and layers of V1 that project to V2 and V4.

The final goal of the connections of color-coded cells in the visual system is to produce responses that correlate with object color constancy and to associate colors with specific objects. The response of cells in V4 agrees with object color constancy. The presence of cells with specificity for borders as well as colors in both V1 and V4 suggests that the shape of an object is analyzed together with its color to provide a unified percept i.e. an orange colored mango or a red apple.

Receptive Fields

Operationally, the receptive field of a neuron is defined as the region in the visual field in which an appropriate stimulus modulates the photoreceptor cell's response. In the lab, electrophysiologists frequently connect the amplified output of the implanted microelectrode monitoring the active neuron to a loudspeaker. This enables them to actually *hear* the differences in crackling sounds emitted by the firing neuron (evoked potential) during the experiment.

Depending on the profile of this auditory cue, numerous types of receptor cells have been discovered in the visual cortex, mediating the quality and intensity of the light stimulus impinging upon its field. The receptive field of most retinal ganglion cells possess a spatial antagonistic structure (on-center /off periphery or off-center/on periphery etc.) that constructs an accurate sketch or *line drawing* of the visual field.

This information flows along the 6 cm long optic nerve of each eye and merges with those from the other at the optic chiasm. Here the right/left visual field input undergoes a hemi-field fragmentation (see figure) and heads for the thalamus and LGN. It is the best known of several thalamic nuclei that process visual information.

The LGN is strategically placed between the retina and the cortex. Incoming retinal information is switched over onto a geniculate relay neuron that sends this data onward to the primary visual cortex. The receptive field of the projection cell is nearly identical to that of its input fibers, to such an extent that it is erroneously assumed, by most researchers that no significant transformation of the retinal input occurs here.

The forward projection from the LGN to the V1 layer of the cortex is much smaller than the V1 feedback channels. This suggests that the cortex is selectively editing (enhancing or suppressing) the retinal input passing through the LGN. The visual input is

collated into discrete regions and analyzed for shape/size and numerous other constancies previously embedded into the master visual program.

Collateral interneurons then dispatch appropriate "copies" to the limbic system and surrounding nuclei for various emotional/visual memory tagging. These multiple pathways, with over a *million* fibers, carry more than 10 *million* bits of visual information per second. That is faster than your standard landline or online DSL hookup!

By the time, the retinal input enters the nine principal areas of the visual cortex, it has already been broken down into individual *pixels*, if you will, each reflecting minute changes in the visual percept of the binocular field out there. Besides a large projection to the superior colliculus, discussed next, numerous minor pathways access an assorted collection of vision mediating nuclei that evaluate blinking, gaze direction, pupillary size, ambient light and other regulatory functions. Since these nuclei do not have a visual map, they do not play a conscious role in cognition.

About 100,000 ganglion cell axons run from the retina to the superior colliculus (SC) straddling the midbrain. The SC is the most important visual processing center in fish, amphibians, turtles and other reptiles. In primates, much of its function has been usurped by the cortex.

It does however coordinate the fine tracking or pursuit movements of the eyeballs via the extra-ocular muscles and mediate the eye/head movements, orienting responses and vestibulo-ocular reflex (from the inner ear). This helps dampen the constant jiggling of the visual field as you look around and walk at the same time.

Some retinal ganglion cells send their axons directly into the inferior pulvinar nucleus. The rest of the pulvinar receives its visual input via the superior colliculus while three of the predominantly visual nuclei project to a wide region of the neocortex including the posterior parietal, the inferior temporal, the prefrontal and orbito-frontal areas.

While the eyes are essential for normal forms of seeing most of the neurons that underlie visual cognition, do not encode eye-of-origin information in an explicit way. They are only concerned with the Big

Picture aspects of your vision and the diverse neuronal structures in the thalamus and cortex read out the optic nerve signals and generate a stable, homogenous and compelling view of the world out there.

The Optic Nerve

Functionally the optic nerve begins at the ganglion cells of the retina. The axons arising from these cells course toward the exit of the optic nerve through the orbit into the skull cavity. From the nasal side, the axons take a straight course toward the optic disc in a sort of funnel-shaped configuration.

The smaller diameter axons from the macular region consolidate into the papillo-macular bundle, which enters the temporal sector of the nerve head. Axons from the rest of the retina follow an arcuate course around the papillo-macular bundle to enter the optic nerve head at the superior and inferior poles. The retinal nerve fiber layer is thickest in these arcuate bundles.

The optic nerve is generally broken up into four segments for ease of description: the intra-ocular (nerve-head, disc and papilla), the intra-orbital, the intra-canalicular (within the optic canal) and a small intra-cranial portion that merges into the optic chiasm and optic tract. Before entering the brain, each optic nerve splits into two parts. The temporal or lateral branch continues to traverse along the same (ipsilateral) side. The nasal or medial branch crosses over to project to the opposite (contralateral) side.

The crossover point is known as the *optic chiasm*. Given the optics of the eye, this crossover of nasal fibers ensures that visual information from each aspect of the visual field is projected to contralateral brain structures. For example, because of the retinal curvature, light reflecting off objects in the *left* visual field is depicted in the temporal retina of the right eye, while the nasal retina of the right eye sees the *right* visual field.

By this crossover mechanism, visual information from the *entire* left field is now conducted to the right visual cortex and vice versa for the other eye making it a lot easier to process binocular information in the brain.

Once inside the brain, each optic nerve divides into pathways that differ with respect to where they terminate within the subcortex. The main pathway to the LGN of the thalamus contains more than 90% of the optic nerve fibers and provides input to the cortex via the geniculo-cortical projections.

The remaining 10% of the fibers innervate other subcortical structures like the pulvinar nucleus of the thalamus and the superior colliculus of the midbrain. However, this apparent paucity of innervation does not, in any way, mean that these pathways are unimportant. The human optic nerve is so large that its 10% constitutes more fibers than are found in the entire auditory pathway.

By this pathway, the one million-odd axons comprising each optic nerve conduct partially processed visual information from the retinal ganglion cells to the LGN, superior colliculus, hypothalamus and various midbrain centers. They are unmyelinated while in the retina and optic nerve-head and gain a sheath only after passing through the *lamina cribrosa* (a multilayered bony sieve).

Fibers from the temporal and nasal retina retain their relative positions in the nerve. The macular fibers occupy of the cross-sectional diameter of the nerve without forming a discrete bundle. As the nerve approaches the chiasma there is some rotation and crossed fibers from the opposite eye may sweep slightly into the nerve. By virtue of this decussation, the right and left hemi-fields of vision are represented in separate cerebral hemispheres. The fibers are now known as the optic tracts.

About 20-30% of fibers leave the optic tract and proceed to the pupillary centers. A virtual vertical line running through each fovea splits the fibers from each hemi-retina. Some overlap of naso-temporal ganglion cells occurs from a 1^0 strip projecting to either hemisphere. This phenomenon is thought to play a role in mediating stereoscopic vision in primates.

The Thalamus & LGN

Thalamus is Greek for "inner chamber" as it lies deep within the brain and was originally thought to be *hollow*. It is in actuality a small egg-shaped structure that rests atop the midbrain and serves as a gateway to the cortex. Both the thalamus and the neocortex evolved in close relationship to each other and are interconnected with profusely branched short and long-reach connections.

The two thalami, one in each hemisphere, are divided into discrete nuclei (cluster of neural networks), each with its own separate input/output channels. Specific nuclei send somatosensory, auditory, visceral and optical information to various relevant cortical and sub-cortical regions. Not only is the thalamus involved in relaying primary sensory information but it also receives input from the basal ganglia, cerebellum, neocortex and the medial temporal lobe.

Two major cholinergic pathways originate in the brainstem and in the basal forebrain. The brainstem cells send an ascending projection to the thalamus, where release of Ach (acetylcholine) facilitates the relay of information from the sensory periphery to the cortex. Cholinergic cells are therefore well positioned to influence the entire cortex by controlling the thalamus. In contrast, cholinergic basal forebrain neurons send their axons to a much wider array of target structures, innervating the thalamus, hippocampus, amygdala and cerebral cortex.

As we shall see in much more detail later on in the discussion on consciousness, cholinergic mechanisms tend to fluctuate with the sleep-wake cycle. In general, much neurological pathology whose symptoms include disturbances of consciousness, such as Parkinson's dss, Alzheimer's

71

and various forms of dementia are associated with a selective loss of cholinergic neurons. The bottom line is that without the ascending influence of the brainstem and thalamic nuclei, an organism cannot be conscious of anything.

By far the best explored of the thalamic nuclei is the lateral geniculate nucleus (LGN). As noted above, the 90% optic nerve fibers terminating in the LGN project in a highly organized manner. The most striking anatomic feature of the LGN is its laminated appearance, which subserves three important properties.

First, three of its layers receive input from one retina while the other three from the other. Ganglion cell axons from the *right* temporal hemi-retina terminate in layers 2,3 and 5 of the *right* LGN while layers 1,4 and 6 serve as terminals for the *left* nasal hemi-retina. The opposite pattern is seen for the left LGN.

(Author's note: It is important to keep in mind that the ipsilateral temporal hemi-retina and contralateral nasal hemi-retina are responsive to the same visual field. This ensures that visual information from a region in space is projected to the same LGN.)

The second organizational principle pertains to the specificity of projections from the visual field to the LGN. Each layer of the LGN contains a topographic map of the retina and thus of external space that is in tight register i.e. an object at a certain location in space will activate cells within each layer that fall along a line perpendicular to the LGN surface. The activation occurs in all six layers.

The third organizing principle reveals that the cell types of each layer have clear distinctions: the bottom two layers contain large (magnocellular) cells whereas the top four has smaller (parvocellular) ones. There are many more parvocellular cells than magnocellular ones. Parvocellular cells represent the world at a fine grain. They also mediate color. A sub-category is red-green opponent cells that receive inputs from L cones in the central, excitatory part of their receptive field and opposing input from M cones in their surround.

Complementary cells are driven by a greenish spot of light directed at their center and are inhibited by a reddish annulus. The magnocellular neurons are much less sensitive to wavelength and have no color opponency organization to speak of. They carry a signal related to the intensity or luminosity (with L, M and S cone contributions).

A striking feature of these pathways is their anatomical independence. Eliminating the parvocellular layers profoundly affects color and high fidelity spatial vision but sensitivity to patterns that morph rapidly with time remain intact. This situation is reversed with destruction of the magnocellular pathways.

Closer inspection reveals a further substructure sandwiched between these two, consisting of small, cone-shaped koniocellular neurons. The koniocellular neurons lack a pronounced, spatial center-surround organization, signaling chromatic opponency instead, i.e. they respond to the difference between S cones and the sum of L and M cones. The visual environment is mapped in a continuous manner onto all geniculate layers.

Visual information is segregated into distinct pathways in the adjacent cortical area called the prestriate cortex or V2. There is a vast amount of cross talk among the P and M cells after the first few synapses in the cortex. Upwards of 30 distinct cortical visual areas have been identified in the macaque. A primary physiological method for establishing such areas is to measure how spatial information is represented across a region of cortex.

Each visual area has a topographic representation of external space in the contralateral hemi-field and the boundaries them are marked by topographical discontinuities. Similar to the LGN, the cortex has at least as many retinotopic maps as visual areas so that topological integrity is preserved.

Although each visual area provides a map of external space, the maps differ in the type of information they represent. For instance, neurons in some areas are highly sensitive to color variation whereas in others they may be sensitive to motion. Rather than each area representing all attributes of an object, each provides its own limited analysis.

As we advance through the visual system, various areas elaborate on the initial information in V1 and begin to integrate this information across dimensions to form recognizable percepts. Researchers labeled the area activated in the color foci as V4 and motion as V5. Because of the convoluted nature of the human visual cortex, a flat representation is constructed.

High-resolution anatomical MRI scans are obtained and computer algorithms are employed to transform the folded, cortical surface into a 2D map by tracing the gray matter. The activation signals from the fMRI study are then plotted on the flattened map with color-coding used to indicate areas that were activated at similar times.

Such imaging studies have aided the analysis of visual illusion phenomena and patterns of brain activation during illusory states can be compared with those observed during visual stimulation. In this way, areas of overlap can provide insight into the level of processing in which illusions arise as well as indicate how information is represented in different visual areas. Results suggest that perception involves higher visual areas rather than the primary visual cortex.

One of the largest thalamic nuclei is called the *pulvinar* and phylogenetically, it is the most recent addition to the thalamus. It is located at the posterior pole of the thalamus and appears as a relatively small but rather well defined cluster in carnivores, increasing progressively in size from monkeys and apes to humans.

It is rather large in humans and has at least three separate visual maps. Unlike the cortex, these maps are not interconnected but stand-alone. They mediate the highly complex areas of vigilance, attention and goal-directed visuo-motor behaviors, most notably in the eye movement area. The visual maps engage when the animal is actively scanning the foliage for predators or prey and switch around rapidly when evaluating the next course of action.

The neurons in these thalamic nuclei fall into two broad classes: excitatory projection cells that send their axons to the cortex and local inhibitory interneurons that fine tune or enhance performance. The projection neurons are subdivided into core and matrix regiments. The core cells aggregate in clusters and target precisely delineated recipient zones in the intermediate layers of various cortical regions.

They are in an ideal position to disperse and help synchronize activity or to provide timing signals to large populations of cells. While the core conveys specific information to its cortical recipients, the matrix might help assemble the widespread neuronal coalitions that mediate the multi-faceted aspects of any conscious percept.

A final note is that the sensory relay nuclei of the thalamus not only project axons to the cortex but also receive heavy descending projections back from the same cortical area they contact. This descending cortico-thalamic projection terminates in a thin layer of cells that surrounds the thalamic nuclei known as the thalamic reticular nucleus.

The neurons in this nucleus form a lateral inhibitory network of cells that may act in the modulation of thalamo-cortical outputs perhaps to fine tune sensory transmission or partially gate the flow of information to the cortex. This structure is not a single nucleus but rather an amorphous conglomeration of several nuclei that interact with the specific thalamic subdivisions they overlay.

The Primary Visual Cortex or V1

The cerebral cortex can be subdivided into the phylogenetically older olfactory (smell) and hippocampus (memory) cortex and the newer neocortex. This multilayered "cake-like" structure crowning the rest of the brain is only found in mammals. The human neocortex and its diverse connections occupy about 80% of the total brain volume. Quite different from other brain structures such as the thalami, basal ganglia or brainstem, the neocortex is a vast *sheet* of neural tissue.

It is highly convoluted and possesses a laminated substructure. The size of one cortical sheet varies across species, ranging from around 1 cm^2 in the tree shrew to about 100 cm^2 in the macaque monkey, 1000 cm^2 in humans and dolphins to several times larger in certain whales. Think of its crinkly appearance as 2 thick pancakes, 35 cm in diameter, crumpled up and stuffed into your skull. The exact pattern of cortical indentations (gyri and sulci) is as unique as an individual fingerprint.

There are many types of cortical neurons. Based on the laminar position of the cell body, dendritic morphology and axonal target zones, about a 100 cell types can be distinguished. Pyramidal cells tend to predominate with extensive inter-connections both inside and outside the cortex.

While the receptive field structure of retinal and geniculate cells is relatively stereotypical, the cortical cells display an amazing variety of selective responses to motion, color, orientation, depth and other stimulus features. Their non-classical receptive field extends far beyond the confines of the region in space that directly excites the cell. It provides the context within which any single visual stimulus is placed.

In humans, much of V1 is buried within the calcarine fissure on the medial wall of the brain as corresponds to Brodmann's area 17. The location and orientation of this fissure can vary between individual brains and the outside world is mapped onto V1 in a topographic manner with neighboring locations in the visual field projecting onto nearby locations. Optometrists refer to this spatial organization as a *retinotopic* map.

The visual cortex contains multiple, superimposed charts or maps for the position, orientation and direction of motion of stimuli, ocular dominance and color. Are these maps related in some way to each other or are they random? It is unclear at this point. What is clear is that visual processing along these two new pathways is designed to extract fundamentally different types of information.

The ventral or occipito-temporal pathway is specialized for object perception and recognition for determining what it is we are looking at. The dorsal or occipito-parietal pathway, on the other hand, is specialized for spatial configuration between different objects in a scene.

"What?" and "Where?" are the two basic questions to be answered in visual perception. Not only must we recognize what we are looking at but also we need to know where it is in order to respond appropriately.

Upon emerging from V1 – and now known as the vision-for-perception (ventral) and the vision-for-action (dorsal) streams – they flow toward the prefrontal cortex.

The ventral stream passes through V2 and V4 into IT and projects from there into the ventrolateral prefrontal cortex. This pathway is responsible for the analysis of form, contour, color, detecting and evaluating objects. The inferior temporal (IT) cortex and associated regions have been implicated in conscious visual perception.

The dorsal pathway moves from V1 through MT and into the posterior parietal (PP) cortex. From there it sends a far-flung projection into the dorsolateral prefrontal cortex. These neurons are concerned with space, motion and depth. It processes visuo-spatial cues necessary for reaching and guiding the eye, hand or arm to appropriate destinations.

Both streams have extensive inter-connections and cross linkages. Some areas, particularly in and around the superior temporal cortex lie at the interface between the two pathways and defy any simple classification.

Beyond V1

The primary visual cortex represents the world in multiple low and high-resolution maps. These emphasize canonical image features such as orientation, changes in image, wavelength-specific information and local depth. Yet it is but the first cortical area of many discovered to date that subserve vision in mammals. In humans, almost 25% of the entire cerebral cortex is known to mediate visual perception and visuo-motor tasks.

Any accessible region of the cortex can be "turned off" by cooling it with metal plates placed on the surface. When V1 is shut down in this manner, visual responses throughout the so-called *ventral hierarchy* are much reduced, so much in some areas that even a basic receptor field is compromised.

However, region MT (middle temporal) that is known to mediate motion processing seems to retain some degree of selectivity for movements. MT is mainly fed by two "tributaries", both of which originate in the retina. One passes through V1 while the other reaches the cortex via the superior colliculus (SC). Consistent with this view is the observation that lesioning the corresponding regions in both V1 and the SC eliminates all responses from MT cells.

This cortical bypass may be adequate to support the minimal, unconscious visuo-motor behavior observed in "blindsight" patients whose V1 has been destroyed but yet insufficient to "power" the ventral pathway for conscious, object vision.

V2, the second visual area encircles V1 and is about equal in size. The neurons from V1 project in a one-to-one correspondence to their counterparts in V2, resulting in a similarly skewed topographic representation there. This mapping extends in a continuous manner across the cortical sheet. There are no abrupt borders but the receptive fields get larger and more diffuse.

The V2 neurons are sensitive to depth, motion, color and form. Many are end-stopped, responding best to short bars, lines or edges. No intensity change is present yet one sees *contours* in the representative visual field defined by either contrast, motion, depth or illusory edges. Its neurons are implicated in identifying partially occluded figures in the visual scene (Where's Waldo?).

Directly adjacent to V2 is a third visual area, V3 with a split mirror-image representation of the visual space, one for the upper and one for the lower field. In front of these are the V3A and V4 areas possessing their own retinotopic map based on inputs from V1, V2 and V3. Its receptive fields are bigger than those of its inputs and the visual information undergoes further evaluation by "fragmentation".

In a series of influential papers, Semir Zeki of University College, London, England suggested that the V4 area mediates color perception in the macaque monkey. Many V4 neurons represent color rather than raw wavelengths of light. However, such color-selective cells are not limited to V4 but present elsewhere in the visual cortex.

In humans, lesions along the ventral surface of the occipital and temporal lobes, part of the fusiform gyrus can selectively disturb color vision i.e. the form and other aspects of vision are present but the hue is gone. This has since been confirmed by fMRI studies done on volunteer subjects.

Intriguingly, some color-tuned regions remain active when subjects experience color after-images in the absence of any physical color. For instance, if you stare for some time at a vivid color (green) and then look at a uniform gray field, you will see its complementary color (red) hang for a short time then fade away. fMRI activity in a section of the fusiform gyrus follows the percept, increasing in response to the virtual color after-image and degrading back to baseline after the inducing color patch has been removed.

In synesthetes, individuals with the unique ability to perceive events in multiple modalities simultaneously i.e. colored-hearing, blind-sight, hearing shapes or seeing touches, hue percepts evoked by words trigger brain activity in the same part of the fusiform gyrus as colored stimuli. Surprisingly, areas V1 and V2 did not show any fMRI response during colored hearing.

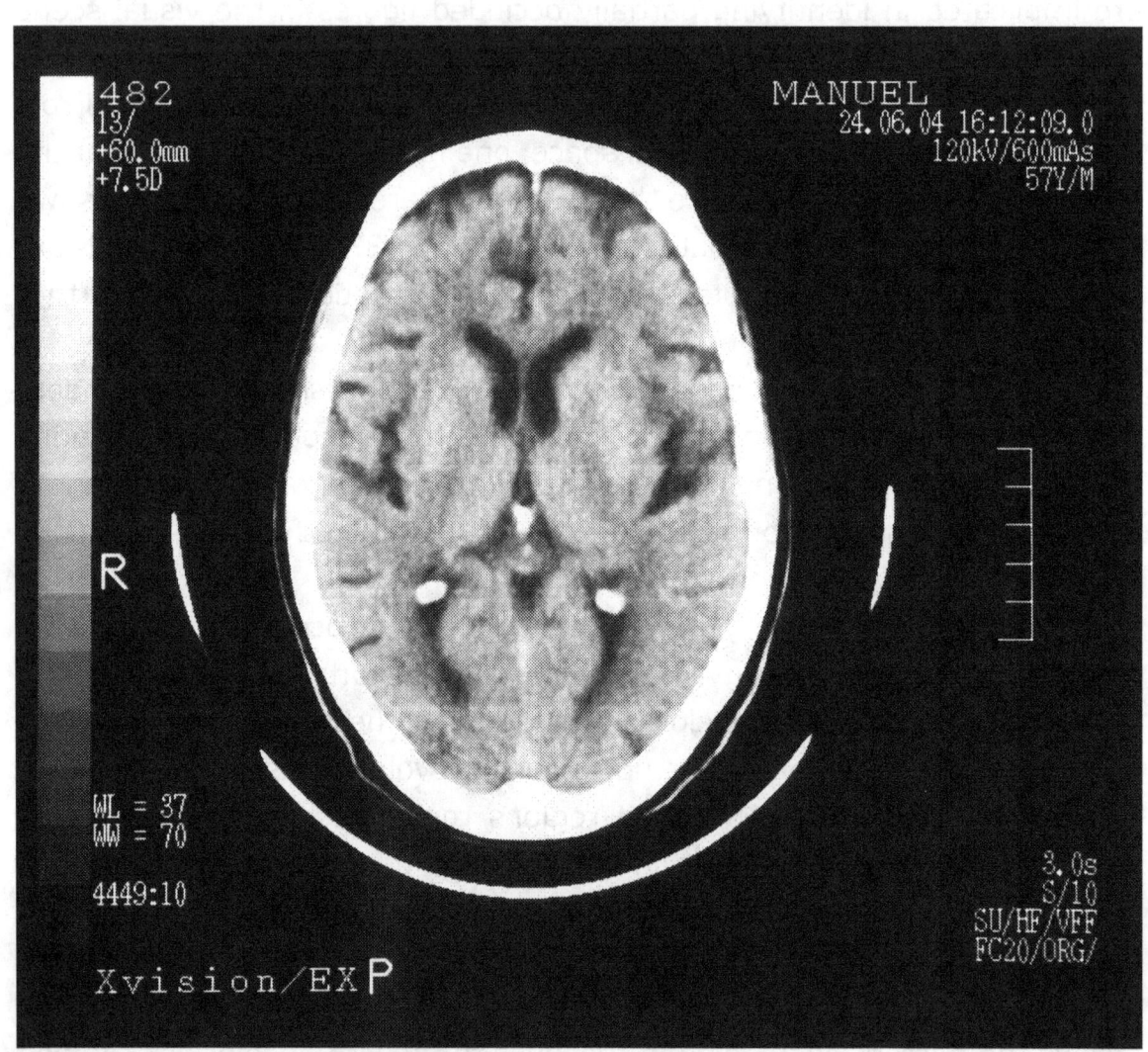

CT scan of Brain: Top View

Brain Maps & Visual Space

The human body's sensory surface and external worlds are represented in cortical maps, which provide a point-for-point representation of neurons responding to visual stimulation. There is a map for the hands, face, torso and each extremity. The higher the resolution a sensory surface has, the more neurons there are to represent that area. For instance, the neurons that respond to fingertips are greater in number and more densely packed than the ones responding to the back of the hand making them more sensitive to touch. This phenomenon is known as the *cortical magnification factor*.

The body maps also seem to follow a logical sequence where the neurons coding for the index finger are situated next to the middle finger, next to the ring finger etc. This is known as somatotopy and such cortical maps are called somatotopic maps. The maps are present in all adult animals and humans and appear to be the basis for the ordering of our perceptions. They reflect the receptive field properties of cortical neurons.

Single-cell recording studies have provided physiologists with a powerful tool to map out the visual areas in the macaque monkey brain and characterize the functional properties of the neurons within them. This work has also provided strong evidence that different visual areas are specialized to represent distinct attributes of the visual scene. Inspired by these results, researchers have employed neuro-imaging techniques to ask whether a similar architecture can be discerned in the human brain.

Semir Zeki of University College in London used PET (positron emission tomography) to verify that different visual areas are activated when subjects are processing color or motion information. Subtractive logic factored out the difference in the activation modes in the control and experimental situations. The results of the two studies provided clear evidence that the two tasks activated distinct brain regions.

Although the spatial resolution of PET is coarse, these areas were determined to be in front of the striate (V1) and prestriate cortex (V2). In contrast, after the appropriate subtraction in the motion experiment, the residual foci were bilateral but near the junction of the temporal, parietal and occipital cortices. These foci were more superior and much more lateral than the ones for color. They were labeled as human V4 for the *color* foci and V5 for the *motion* task (most researchers now refer to this area as human MT even though it is not in the temporal lobe of the human brain).

The activation maps in this PET study are rather crude. More recently, sophisticated functional magnetic resonance imaging (fMRI) techniques have been applied to study the organization of the human brain and visual cortex in particular. In these studies, a stimulus is systematically moved across the visual field. The blood oxygen level dependent (BOLD) response for areas representing the superior quadrant will tend to increase at a different time than the response for areas representing the inferior quadrant, allowing the entire field to be continuously tracked.

In order to compare areas that respond to foveal stimulation and those that respond to peripheral stimulation, a dilating and contracting ring stimulus is used. By combining these different stimuli, researchers can measure the cortical representation of the contralateral visual field.

Because of the convoluted nature of the human visual cortex, the results from such an experiment would be indecipherable if we were to plot the data on the anatomical maps found in a brain atlas. To avoid this problem, a flat representation is constructed. High-resolution anatomical MRI scans are obtained and computer algorithms are employed to transform the folded, cortical surface into a two-dimensional map by tracing the gray matter.

The activation signals from the fMRI study are then plotted on the flattened map, with color-coding used to indicate areas that were activated at similar times. Boundaries between visual areas are defined by reversals in the retinotopic representation within a quadrant and the foveal regions are well identified by a string of asterisks.

A number of maps encode object position (location) using implicit representations that depend on the actuator concerned. Thus, the eye movement system contains a different representation of visual space than the brain region encoding visually guided reach movements.

Some neurons do explicitly encode object location in the brain. So-called *place* cells have been isolated from the rodent hippocampus, which fire maximally when the animal is physically within a particular region in its environment. These neurons remain silent outside this restricted area.

Functional imaging of the human brain has revealed object-specific zones in the cortex. The sight of objects selectively activates the ventral temporal (VT) cortex, including the *fusiform gyrus* and the lateral occipital region. Most researchers agree that the sight of human faces preferentially activates the so-called fusiform *face* area (FFA) in the fusiform gyrus. Induced lesions in this neighborhood are often associated with an inability to recognize faces.

Currently, a debate rages between localists who assign one chunk of the ventral stream to the dedicated analysis of faces, another one to body parts, a third sector to houses and spatial scenes. Holists argue that object recognition is more widely distributed in patches of overlapping activity throughout the brain.

Independent or Convergent Pathways

Thus far, we have emphasized that the visual system contains multiple pathways; each specialized to extract specific information. Yet the outputs from these pathways are designed to complement each other. This paradox has resulted in a lively debate concerning the inherent independence of such pathways. Advocates favoring a segregationist viewpoint focus on anatomical, physiological and behavioral data. They indicate that the processing of features such as motion and color involve separable mechanisms from the first synapse in the CNS all the way to the extrastriate cortex. To these theorists, neurological dissociations are the crowning piece of evidence.

On the other side are those who emphasize the lack of perfect segregation. Cells in the M and P-blob pathways exhibit some orientation selectivity. Color sensitivity is not the exclusive domain of the P-blob pathway but also found in the P-interblob ones. Lesion studies of animals have also brought into question the notion that the processing of features like depth, color and orientation depends solely on a single pathway.

For these reasons, the term concurrent processing was coined by David Van Essen, which emphasizes the analytical characteristics of visual perception. As noted from the foregoing discussion on PET imaging, there is strong evidence that the visual system does not analyze the input *en masse* but breaks it up into its various constituents (line drawings or sketches) and then builds up the *gestalt* or global percept of the visual scene.

Tactile "Seeing"

At present it is unclear how tactile information ends up activating the visual cortical neurons in blind people. One possibility is that a massive reorganization of cortico-cortical connections follows peripheral blindness. The sensory-deprived visual cortex is taken over, perhaps through back projections originating in *polymodal* association cortical areas.

This issue was explored in a recent PET study whose results suggest a remarkable degree of cortical plasticity and a neurobiological mechanism. The greater non-visual perceptual acuity exhibited by blind people was first noted by Louis Braille when he was motivated to develop his tactile reading system. He was spurred on by his belief that vision loss was offset by a heightened sensitivity in the fingertips.

One account of this compensation focuses on non-perceptual mechanisms. While the sensory representation of somato-sensory information is similar for blind and sighted subjects, since the former group is not distracted by vision or visual imagery and they may be using the system more efficiently. It is also entirely possible that somatosensory projections to the thalamic relays spread into the nearby LGN, exploiting the now defunct geniculo-striate pathway in the sightless.

Maturation of Subcortical Visual Circuits

The foveal region in the human retina is immature at birth, whereas the peripheral retina is more developed. Hence, newborn vision is driven predominantly by peripheral inputs. In a similar way, the optic nerve is not myelinated completely in the newborn but it proceeds at a rapid pace, reaching adult-like patterns within two years. The LGN, acting as the main relay between the retina and cortex also experiences rapid growth in the first six months, almost doubling in volume.

The primary visual cortex matures in stages, the deeper layers which project to the superior colliculi (SC) developing earlier than the more superficial ones. The SC is the main subcortical target of the retinal ganglion cells and mediates eye movements (oculomotor and saccadic). It is the first subcortical circuit to be myelinated in the visual array and primarily drives the infant visuomotor behavior.

By one month of age, the infant is able to fixate for longer periods. Coincident with this behavior is the development of projections from the striate cortex (V1) to the subcortical structures that inhibit activity in the SC i.e. automatic overt orienting is replaced by selective fixation.

By two months, infants develop smooth pursuits and begin to show normal orienting to novel stimuli presented in the visual field (VF). The infants also begin to attend to the internal features of complex stimuli as their macular region matures leading to enhanced visual acuity. The pattern in smooth pursuit may result from the coincident development and maturation of V1 projections to the middle temporal (MT) motion areas, which pathway is critical for mediating them.

Between three and six months, infants are capable of anticipatory eye movements. This is possible via maturation of projection pathways from the upper layers of V1 to the frontal eye fields responsible for voluntary eye movements. Now their visual acuity reaches normalcy and these infants are able to integrate the two eyes into a binocular percept.

Development of Face Recognition

Facial feature recognition is an exquisitely developed skill in humans that has its origins in the first days of life. Newborns seem to like looking at human faces or face-like stimuli more than they like looking at abstract patterns. Infants just a few weeks old can distinguish their mother's face from other women's faces but since they have such poor visual acuity, they primarily rely on global aspects (smile, hairline etc.) of her facial features.

After 3-4 months of age when their acuity becomes more normal, they are better able to distinguish among various faces and even have a toothy smile for other family members. However, event-related potentials recorded in response to faces suggest that face processing does not fully mature until puberty. Thus although precocial skills are seen in newborns, face processing requires a good deal of experience before it is fully developed.

This early stage of "facial awareness" may be mediated by subcortical pathways, which in turn help to shape the further development of the association cortices to which they send neural projections. Over time, the constant fixation on numerous facial profiles around them and correlated neural activity associated with this behavior "wire-up" the higher-order regions of the brain to process faces in more adult-like patterns. Based on available developmental data, the early precortical stage is relatively short-lived in comparison to the later more protracted adult-like phase of face recognition.

Language Acquisition

Humans are not born with the ability to understand or speak a particular language; they must learn it through exposure and practice. However, humans and some higher primates do possess an innate ability to acquire or learn to speak and understand a language. This may sound semantic but there is an essential difference. For example, let us take human bipedality.

Though our parents guided us in learning to walk as infants, even without any instructions we would eventually stand up and begin to walk. It can be categorized as a normal characteristic of *Homo sapiens* that occurs at a certain stage of human development. Walking has dedicated neural structures and circuits that are common to all humans around the globe. It is an innate ability whereas acquiring a language is not.

That said, most humans also are able to acquire any language during childhood they are exposed to. Some neural structures that mediate the ability to acquire spoken languages like semantics and grammar appear to be subserved by nonidentical neural systems regardless of the speaker's native tongue.

Humans seem to have an innate knowledge of linguistics that enables them to employ syntactic structures of language. They are thus able to develop complex forms of linguistic representation that is part of the human brain's specialization for language.

Some Anomalies of Sensory Neural Integration

Synesthesia

In synesthesia, neural events in one sensory modality induce vivid, lifelike experiences in another. For example, synesthetes perceive written words or numbers in full color; geometric shapes take on different flavors or sounds and touched body-parts lead to psychedelic visual *auras*.

For obvious reasons, many of these gifted individuals are prone to hiding their 'affliction'. However, it is estimated that at least one in a thousand has this special ability. It tends to run in families, is *six* times more common in females, shows preference for left-handers and especially prevalent in writers, poets and artists (the so-called *right brain* people).

Studies have shown that these experiences cannot be consciously suppressed and indicate that the perceptions of such synesthetes are indeed real and not confabulations of an overactive imagination. Some recent work performed by neuroscientists, implicate discrete areas of the *Limbic System* and the 'emotional health' of the individual as playing a prominent role in their mediation.

Multisensory integration within the CNS depends on each individual neuron responding to input from more than one sensory modality. In most of us, however, the senses remain isolated and easily distinguishable i.e. very rarely are we 'confused' as to what we are really seeing, hearing or touching. Primates usually construct a spatial map of their surroundings in order to better 'navigate' through the neighborhood.

In humans, information from the 'five' senses are coordinated and projected to the *superior colliculus* of the midbrain, where it is collated

Nazir Brelvi, OD

to produce a 3D map of the space out there. When information from various sensory modalities emanate from the same location in the outside world, the resulting integration leads to a superior 'understanding' of the presenting situation, leading to an appropriate response by the perceiving individual.

Blindsight

It is quite possible that when elaborate visual systems evolved in humans, cortical areas subsumed functions that had depended on subcortical areas in our ancestors. Within the cortical pathways, humans and other primates exhibit a functional division between regions devoted to representing spatial information ("where" processing) and regions devoted to object recognition or "what" processing.

Nonetheless, the subcortical visual pathways in humans do appear to mediate spatial orientation. Evidence for this has come from intriguing studies involving patients who have suffered lesions in the visual cortex inducing cortical blindness. The patient acts and feels as if he is blind yet shows a residual ability to localize stimuli.

While the so-called blindsight phenomenon has been reported in Neurological literature for decades, the interpretation of the effect remains controversial. It may well turn out that different aspects of it are attributable to different mechanisms. It is possible that information can reach extrastriate visual areas in the cortex either through direct geniculate projections or via projections from other subcortical structures.

Another possibility could be that the lesions in the primary cortex are "shallow" and that blindsight results from residual (subliminal?) function in the spared tissue i.e. the representations in the damaged region of the cortex may be sufficient to guide eye movements (intact Edinger Westphal nucleus?), even though the patients fail to achieve awareness.

Nonetheless, an important feature of many blindsight studies is that patients can localize stimuli they are not aware of. This ability to orient toward a stimulus fits the known functions of the retino-collicular pathway.

The superior and inferior colliculi receive input from the visual and auditory pathways respectively. They use it to construct a representation of where objects are in visual or auditory space and to guide the eyes to them.

As an object is detected on the margins of the visual field, the retino-collicular pathways are activated that "order" the eyes to move and foveate the object of interest. From this view, we might expect that stimulus falling within the scotoma (of a hemianopic patient, for instance) would activate the collicular activating system.

In a clever test of this hypothesis, Robert Rafal measured how quickly patients with dense scotomas could look at stimuli presented in their *intact* visual field. Since the patients were conscious of the stimuli, the task seemed quite reasonable. However, Rafal also presented a simultaneous stimulus to the scotomatous region, which the patient did not report seeing.

Nonetheless, the irrelevant stimuli led to a significant boost in patient reaction time on comparison to normal situations when the stimuli were only presented to the intact visual field. Through this implicit measure of interference, we see evidence of residual processing within scotomas. Rafal and associates suggested that this interference arises from the irrelevant stimulus providing a competing activation in the intact retino-collicular pathway and that this competition slows eye movement toward the target.

Further evidence that this interference is related to the collicular system comes from a second experiment where subjects were asked to press a button after detecting the target rather than look at it. Now the competing stimuli had no effect on reaction time.

Thus, the interference was present only when the response required an eye movement, a result that meshes with the functions of the superior colliculus. It appears that a collicular orienting system remains intact in hemianopic patients with lesions restricted to the primary visual cortex.

Binocular Vision

Just because we have two eyes does not mean that we possess binocularity. There are quite a few mammals and birds with overlapping visual fields that are not truly fulltime binocular like the primates. Each eyeball needs to be wired into the visual cortex in a special way for the brain to fuse the retinal 'images' into a stereoscopic whole.

We know this because about two percent of the population can see well with each eye individually but the random-dot stereograms (a test of binocularity or stereopsis) remain flat. Another small percent possess poor degrees of stereopsis ranging from intermittent to flat fusion. This variety of 'stereo-blindness' appear to be genetically determined, suggesting that the visual cortex is 'assembled' piecemeal and not as a complete module.

Stereovision is not present at birth and can be permanently damaged in children or young animals if even one of the eyes is temporarily deprived of sight for a few days. When infants are born every neuron in the receiving layer of the visual cortex "adds up" the inputs from corresponding locations in the two eyes rather than keep them separate. The brain is unable to form a right-left spatial map of each eye individually.

Around the two to three month stage, the visual cortex becomes sophisticated enough to differentiate from which eye the input is originating. As soon as this happens, a sort of "rivalry" occurs between the two eyes as their spatial maps now have a built-in bias. Each eye is interpreting a different aspect of the visual field with a large central area of 'overlap'. This mismatch called *binocular rivalry* forms the basis of random-dot acuity in primates.

Once the brain has segregated the left eye's image from the right eye's, subsequent layers of neurons can compare them for the minute disparities that signal depth. When the random dot pattern, usually generated by a computer, is seen by the viewer, the tiny disparities built into the pattern are interpreted by the brain as a picture containing various degrees of depth i.e. three dimensions rather than just two.

Suddenly, as the numerous inputs to the visual cortex coalesce the flat 2D dotted image begins to morph *magically* into a robust 3D one, sometimes so rapidly that the viewer may take a step back or bob his head around in curious surprise.

Just as Hollywood makes use of the *persistence* of vision to convert flashing still pictures into movies, this peculiarity of the visual system is exploited in the various Magic eye pictures and so called "optical illusions" like the Necker Cube, mother-daughter, vase-human face profiles etc. popularized in sundry magazines/books.

Stereovision is information processing that we experience as a particular flavor of consciousness, a subtle connection between mental computation and awareness. Even

mediated by the extra-ocular and ciliary muscles of the two eyes, it is sensitive to

experience. That is why, if you have seen a certain stereogram before, the image pops out instantly and gets more detailed as you scrutinize it.

The discoveries regarding this 'tunability' of stereopsis in different species affords a novel way of thinking about learning in general. According to Steven Pinker of MIT:

"Learning is often described as an indispensable shaper of amorphous brain tissue. Instead it might be an innate adaptation to the project-scheduling demands of a self-assembling animal". In other words, Pinker feels that the genome builds as much of the organism as possible but leaves the final details of physical development to an information-gathering mechanism.

Several brain researchers have found that this fine-tuning of the neocortex occurs at the local level (lateral geniculate body/ superior colliculus) where the receptor organ (eye) is 'hardwired' to the brain as and when needed during development. This process may have evolved in response to identifiable selection pressures in the ecology of our ancestors.

It provides *reasonable* solutions to unsolvable problems by making tacit assumptions about the world out there.

Most neuroscientists recognize that at the highest levels of cognition, we consciously plod through various steps and invoke rules we learned in school or discovered ourselves. The 'mind' is compared to a complex production system with symbolic inscriptions embedded in a huge memory bank with a bevy of minions that carry out the procedures. At a lower level, the inscriptions and rules are implemented in minor neural networks, which respond to familiar patterns and associate them with other patterns.

However, the boundary is in dispute. Do simple neural networks handle the bulk of everyday thought, leaving only the products of book learning to be handled by explicit rules and propositions?

On the other hand, are the networks more like building blocks that are not humanly smart until assembled into structured representations and programs?

It is often heard that animals are not well engineered at all. The process of natural selection is hobbled by shortsightedness, the dead hand of the past and crippling constraints on what kinds of structures are biologically and physically possible. Much unlike a human engineer, natural selection is incapable of good design. Animals are clunking jalopies saddled with ancestral junk and more often than not blunder into barely serviceable solutions.

People are so eager to believe this claim that they seldom question the whereabouts of this hypothetical engineer that is not constrained by availability of parts, manufacturing practicality or the inherent laws of physics. Sure natural selection does not have the foresight of engineers but it also dispenses with their impoverished imagination, mental hang-ups or rabid conformity to *bourgeois* sensibilities and stakes in profitability.

Guided only by whatever works, the relentless process of natural selection can invent brilliant creative solutions. For millennia, biologists have delighted in the ingenious contrivances found in the animal world: the biomechanical perfection of cheetahs, the infrared sensors of snakes, the ultrasound echolocation apparatus of bats and dolphins, the superglue of marine barnacles, and the super strong silk of spiders, the prehensile tails of macaques or the manual dexterity of humans.

After all, entropy and the more malevolent forces of nature are constantly gnawing at an organism's right to survive, culling the herd with relentless impunity and avidly decimating the outcomes of sloppy engineering. Gould has emphasized that natural selection has only limited freedom to alter basic body plans. Much of the plumbing, wiring and morphology of the primates, for example, have been unchanged for millions of years.

Presumably, they have emerged from embryological 'blueprints' that cannot easily be tinkered with. However, the primate body plan can accommodate marmosets, monkeys, tarsiers, lemurs, chimps, orangs, gorillas and hominids. The similarities are important but so are the differences. Developmental constraints are only able to rule out broad classes of options. They cannot induce a fully functional organ to come into being.

Natural selection can only pick–n-choose from alternatives that are growable as carbon-based living stuff. Another widespread misconception is that if an organ changed its function in the course of evolution, it did not evolve by natural selection. However, a detailed look at the animal world reveals that many organs that we see today have maintained their original function.

For example, the eye was always a visual organ whether it began as a light-sensitive spot or ended up as an eagle eye. Others did change their function. Pectoral fins of fishes became the forelimbs of horses, the flippers of whales, the wings of birds, digging implements of burrowing animals or the brachiating arms of orangutans. More often, before an organ was selected to assume its current job, it was adapted for something else.

The delicate chain of bones forming the middle ear in primates actually began as jawbones in reptiles. Reptiles often sense vibrations by lowering their jaws to the ground. As the mammals came into their own after the devastation of reptiles in the cosmic holocaust of 65 million years ago and began to occupy diverse ecological niches, this function gradually transformed the lower jaw into a much-reduced vibration-sensing organ in mammals. Over millennia, these tiny bones became nestled in the temporal bone forming the middle ear of primates.

There is nothing mysterious about the evolution of bird wings either. Half a wing will not enable you to soar like an eagle but it will let you glide gently from tree to tree or parachute you down from a tall tree to the forest floor, to help cushion your fall. Flapping their vestigial wings do afford ostriches and the lowly chicken to get the hell out of the predator's way in a hurry apart from raising a dust cloud to also foil the cat's evil intentions.

Electrophysiological recordings in the macaque, clinical reports and brain imaging in humans implicate the posterior parietal (PP) cortex in combining and expressing position information and relating it to action. The PP is subdivided into numerous functionally distinct regions where the neuronal responses that are neither purely sensory nor purely motor but a blend of both.

Single-cell experiments indicate the PP is involved in such diverse functions as analyzing spatial relations among objects, controlling eye-hand coordination and determining where to allocate visual attention next. PP is an important conduit for action-related information. The output pathways include direct projections from layer 5 of the PP to the spinal cord, brainstem and reciprocal connections to the premotor and prefrontal areas of the cortex.

Eye Movements & Binocular Disparity

Kinetic Equilibrium Mechanisms

As you weave your way through crowds of commuters in Grand Central Station, your torso, legs and arms continuously adjust themselves so that you remain upright and avoid bumping into anybody. Even though you are quite oblivious of such action corrections, numerous neural networks mediate balance and body posture in real time via continuously updated information from many modalities, not just vision.

By just looking carefully at the various animals we can see that eye positions change from a lateral aspect where each eye is visualizing its own panorama, to eyes with higher degrees of overlapping fields. When the eyes are in the primary position of gaze i.e. viewing objects at optical infinity, the binocular field can be considered as simply the amount of overlap of each monocular field.

For front-facing eyes, the visual axes are almost parallel and the monocular field overlap quite maximum. Some animals possess rather prominent snouts, bills or other facial features that may limit the binocular field. Only simians and humans appear to have developed an ability to converge the eyes so as to bifixate objects as close as a few inches from the bridge of the nose.

The eyes and their distinct patterns of movement are a fascinating source of information. A total of six eye muscles are responsible for rotating the eyeball in several predetermined or learned patterns by the brain. A *saccade* is a rapid (usually measured in milliseconds) movement of both eyes yoked together to "zoom" in on an object of interest. *Pursuits*, on the other hand, are smooth continuous tracking movements of both eyes used to keep the object of interest in constant view while both the viewer and object are in motion.

When the eye movement is off target (overshoot or undershoot), a corrective saccade of small amplitude is triggered to bring the target back onto the fovea. Contrary to popular opinion, the eyes move all the time even when they are "locked-on" to a target. These tiny "jiggles", known as micro-saccades take place within Panum's space (explained in another section). These micro-saccades prevent the retinal image from fading or going away.

The intervals between saccades are brief, as short as 120-130 msec. This corresponds to the minimum time needed to process visual information during fixation. Saccades are usually mediated by the superior colliculi of the brain while the smooth pursuits are coordinated by parietal and/or prefrontal cortex.

If eye movements are prevented or the extra-ocular muscles are tranquilized during surgery, vision rapidly fades into an indistinct "fog". It is often assumed that such "fading to black" is a purely retinal phenomenon caused by the stability of an image on the photoreceptors. Unfortunately, very little is known about the neuronal basis of fading but it may have something to do with the refractory periods of the ganglion cells and the constant need to keep neural impulses flowing through the optic nerve into the LGN to keep the "movie" alive.

The stability and sharpness of the visual world during eye movements is a direct consequence of numerous processes including *saccadic suppression*, a mechanism that interferes with vision during eye movements. This can be experienced by looking in a mirror and fixating each eye alternately. You will never catch your eyes in transition when going back and forth with each eye.

It seems that during the transition phase, vision is partially shut down by the brain. This eliminates blur and the queasy feeling of a world in motion around you. Why then isn't everyday continuous vision "gappy" and broken up by sudden saccades or blinks? Some researchers have postulated the presence of a trans-saccadic integration mechanism that fills in these intervals with a "fictive" movie bridging the retinal images just before and after the blink or saccade.

Nazir Brelvi, OD

The extraocular muscles (EOMs) responsible for moving the eyes receive their innervation from the nuclei of the 3rd, 4th and 6th cranial nerves. The control system coordinates the activity of the alpha motoneurons in these nuclei and premotor networks interconnecting areas in the cerebral cortex and brainstem carry out the task. To enable such coordination, the nuclei are also interconnected by numerous fibers forming the medial longitudinal fasciculus (MLF).

The control system uses sensory information from several sources. For example, the retina informs about whether the image is stationary or slipping in real time, the vestibular nuclei monitoring the degree of head tilt or rotation along the Y & Z axes and the impulses coming from the proprioceptors in the eye muscles relaying information about the actual eyeball coordinates within the orbits. All this sensory information is integrated by the brain and transformed into a single volley of *motor* signals that help fine-tune EOM activity.

There is an important difference between the control of EOMs and other muscles subjected to precise voluntary control e.g., finger movements of a pianist: the nuclei of the EMs, in contrast to the spinal motoneurons, receive no direct fibers from the cerebral cortex. The central control is exerted via premotor networks in the brainstem. In fact, eye movements are voluntary only in a limited sense. We cannot move the two eyes independently of each other like the chameleon and the slow pursuit movements of which we are aware can only be performed when tracking a moving target.

Different central nervous networks control each of the numerous movements that the eyeballs perform every day although all converge on the alpha motoneurons controlling the EOMs. Recent studies show that several regions, for example in the cerebral cortex and the cerebellum participate in the control of both saccadic and pursuit movements.

Signals informing about desired eye position, actual position, retinal slip and position of the head are integrated in the reticular formation (RF) lying adjacent to the eye muscle nuclei in the brainstem. The lateral regions of the pontine nuclei mediate voluntary pursuit movements and the slow-phase components of OKN (optokinetic nystagmus).

Vertical eye movement control mechanisms are found in the mesencephalic RF close to the oculomotor nucleus. The premotor "gaze centers" are supplied by the vestibular nuclei, the superior colliculus, the cerebral cortex and others with relevant information named above. At least two regions of the cerebral cortex are closely involved in the control of EMs: the frontal eye field is primarily related to initiation of saccades whereas several smaller areas in the parieto-temporal region mediate pursuits.

Fusion, Stereopsis & Panum's Space

Normal binocular vision implies binocular single vision (fusion) and a high level of stereoacuity. Stereopsis is the binocular perception of depth enabled by the two eyes viewing the external world from disparate vantage points. The depth estimates in stereoscopic vision are not absolute or egocentric estimates but depend on the fixation point being either nearer or farther away.

Stereoscopic depth perception requires the correlation of visual information from both eyes that are frontally placed to allow a considerable overlap of the binocular visual fields. It also requires yoked eye movements so that the objects stimulate corresponding retinal points and a semi-decussation of the optic tract to permit the interaction of inputs from corresponding regions of each retina. Retinal points in the two eyes are said to be corresponding if *when stimulated separately* they appear to have the *same* visual direction.

The term *horopter*, (Greek *horos*, boundary), defined as the locus of points seen as single with the two eyes was originally introduced by Aguilonius in 1613 to explain the concept of corresponding points in the two retinas having the same monocular visual direction. It was conceived as a surface in visual space. Since that time, the application of the horopter concept has shifted away from a special concern for binocular single vision toward more general problems of stereopsis.

Both, from a theoretical and a physiological point of view, the horopter is best defined as the locus of maximal stereoacuity. In line with this definition, the horopter can also be conceptualized as a zero-disparity reference plane that contains the fixation point and relative to which stereoscopic depth estimates are made.

Wheatstone, by his invention of the stereoscope in 1838, was the first to recognize that disparate retinal images provide the essential cue for binocular depth perception. His idea was basically simple. Take two pictures from slightly different vantage points similar to your two eyes, place the right picture in front of the viewer's right eye and do the same with the left. The brain assuming that the two images are from the real world ends up combining them into a cyclopean image and the binocular parallax provides the three-dimensionality or depth to the percept.

However, as is evident from our earlier discussion on binocular vision, all humans fail to see these stereograms in stereo. Stereovision gives information only about *relative* depth i.e. how much the object of regard is in front or behind the fixation point (plane). This is mediated in the brain by integrating information from the focusing reflex mechanism (ciliary muscle and crystalline lens) and vergence movements (extra-ocular muscles), both of which are yoked.

In order to see the stereogram in full 3D glory, these two mechanisms need to be uncoupled. Viewers resort to various ways to achieve this uncoupling: some cross their eyes at an imaginary distance in front of the stereogram and "free-fuse"; some intentionally view the full picture as if through a mild "fog" by going into a "soft-focus" mode etc.

Another thing Wheatstone recognized was that stimulation of disparate or non-corresponding retinal points could still produce single vision, effectively contradicting the theory of corresponding retinal points.

Panum, in 1858, proposed that the singleness of binocular vision was not confined to a single surface but extended over a volume in space. He argued that for any point on one retina, there is a small *circle* or *area of points* on the other retina, stimulation of which will lead to fusion of two monocular inputs.

Thus, binocular single vision is not limited to the immediate vicinity of the horopter, but extends for a small distance proximal and distal to it. This space came to be known as Panum's fusional area beyond which the subject will see two images (physiological diplopia) of the object rather than just one. Studies show that at the fixation point the extent of Panum's area is approximately 15 minutes of arc, well within the normal range of the human foveola. These results are also similar to those inferred from studies of fixation disparity.

Fixation disparity is a variant of normal binocular vision. The disparities are usually found to be small, ranging from -5 to +3 minutes of arc. In any case, they cannot be larger than Panum's fusional area if diplopia is not to result. Furthermore, they found that the extent of the fusional area was the same for vertical or horizontal disparities.

The extent of Panum's fusional area increases with increasing eccentricity away from the fixation point. Interestingly, Panum's area depends greatly on the class of stimulus and upon achieving binocularly; stabilized global stereopsis may stretch to almost 2^0 in the horizontal direction without loss of stereopsis or fusion. It seems therefore that there is a fairly large tolerance for disparate images once fusion has been obtained.

Binocular Rivalry

Consider the twelve lines making up the Necker cube. Due to the inherent ambiguity of inferring its 3D shape from a 2D drawing on a plane sheet of paper, the lines of the cube can be interpreted in two ways, each differing in their *orientation* in space. Without perspective and shading cues, *either* percept is possible. Even though the line drawing does not change, conscious perception does flip back and forth between the two interpretations in what is known as a *bistable* percept.

Interestingly, you never see the cube suspended in space, halfway in either of the two positions nor do you see a blend of the two figures. Your mind cannot simultaneously visualize both shapes. Instead, each configuration vies for perceptual dominance. This is but one manifestation of a general phenomenon that in the presence of ambiguity prefers to accept a single interpretation, which may change with time. This aspect of experience is sometimes referred to as the unity of consciousness.

In the course of everyday life, your eyes are constantly presented with similar but non-identical views of the world. The brain can extract sufficient cues from the small discrepancies between these two images to discern depth. Lets take another example from Optometry called the Worth's Four Dot. Here, the subject dons a pair of red-green glasses and views a flashlight with two red dots at the 3 and 9 o'clock positions and a green dot at the 12 o'clock position. The 6 o'clock position has a clear dot.

When the subject is asked to report the color of the 6 o'clock clear dot, they invariably report a red or green dot depending on which of their eyes is dominant or an alternating red-green configuration or a yellowish dot if unable to decide. The two red-green percepts tend to alternate in this manner indefinitely but only one is seen while the other is suppressed.

During this so-called binocular rivalry, the two enter and depart from consciousness in a never-ending dance. What you see is not a superposition or blending of the two images but just one. It may belong to the dominant eye, which the brain uses preferentially for most viewing tasks. The duration of these dominance periods i.e. how long either one is visible, varies considerably across subjects and trials.

Binocular rivalry can be thought of as a reflexive alternation between percepts that can be influenced though not completely abolished by sensory or cognitive factors. At the neuronal level, rivalry was long believed to be due to reciprocal inhibition between populations of cells representing input from the left and from the right eyes. One coalition fires away, preventing the other from responding. As this inhibition fatigues, the other group eventually dominates.

Recent psychological and imaging evidence has suggested that this automatic switching is complemented by active processes linked to attention. Mechanisms located in prefrontal and parietal areas can bias the system toward one or the other coalition. This enables the chosen coalition to build up sufficient strength to dominate and to widely distribute its informational content, bringing that image to consciousness.

Where in the brain does the fight for dominance occur?

The retinal neurons are not influenced by the percept. They are driven exclusively by the photoreceptor input. Perceptual modulation could occur as early as the lateral geniculate nucleus, halfway between the retina and primary visual cortex. However, recordings from geniculate neurons have shown that their firing rate is indifferent to whether a monkey saw a rivalrous or a non-rivalrous stimulus. The interplay between dominant and suppressed stimuli, therefore, occurs in the cortex.

The cortical sites underlying binocular rivalry in monkeys were explored by numerous researchers, at MIT and elsewhere. They found that the majority of cells in the primary (V1) and secondary (V2, V4 etc.) visual cortices fired with little regard for the ebb and flow of perception. Largely, a neuron increased its activity to the stimulus in one eye no matter what the macaque monkey saw.

Only six of the 33 cells were somewhat modulated by perception. The majority of V1 cells fire no matter whether the monkey sees one or the other stimuli. This implies that exuberant cortical activity does not guarantee a conscious percept i.e. not just any cortical activity contributes to consciousness.

What about intermediate cortical areas? Do they mediate binocular rivalry?

The neuronal response patterns in areas V4 and MT are more varied than those in V1. About 40% of V4 cells are correlated with the animal's behavior, that is, with its (assumed) perception. The firing profile of many of these cells indicates that they change their output primarily during transitions when the percept changes over from one image to another.

One plausible conclusion is that the coalitions in these intermediate cortical areas are competing against each other attempting to resolve the ambiguity imposed by the two disparate images. At some point, the winner is established and its identity (and probably that of the loser) is signaled to the next stages of visual analysis.

When the researchers recorded from cells in the inferior temporal (IT) cortex and in the lower bank of the superior temporal sulcus (STS), that delimits IT on its upper side; they found that the competition between the rivalrous stimuli was resolved. Nine out of ten cells fired in congruence with the macaque's percept i.e. whenever the monkey saw the preferred image, the neuron fired. When the other image dominated, the cell was mute. Unlike the situation in V4 and MT, no IT cells signaled the suppressed and invisible image.

The IT cortex and neighboring regions not only project to the prefrontal cortex but also receive input from it. What is the role of this feedback in binocular rivalry and related phenomena?

To explore these questions, Nikos Logothetis of the Max Planck Institute turned to the analysis of binocular rivalry in macaques. He trained his monkeys to press one of two levers to indicate which object was being perceived. To ensure that the monkeys were not responding randomly, he included non-rivalrous trials in which only one of the objects was presented.

Recordings were then made from single cells in various areas of the visual cortex. Within each area, he would select two objects, only one of which was effective in driving the cell. In this way, he could correlate the activity of the cell with the animal's perceptual experience.

As his recordings moved up the ventral pathway, Logothetis found an increase in the percentage of active cells, with activity mirroring the animal's perception rather than the stimulus conditions. In V1, the responses of less than 20% of the cells fluctuated as a function of whether the monkey perceived the effective or ineffective stimulus. In V4, this percentage increased to over 33%.

In contrast, the activity of all cells in the visual areas of the temporal lobe was tightly correlated with the animal's perception. Here the cells would respond only when the effective stimulus was perceived. When the monkey pressed the lever indicating that it perceived the ineffective stimulus under rivalrous conditions, the cells were essentially silent.

In both V4 and the temporal lobe, the change in cell activity occurred in advance of the animal's response that the percept had changed. Thus, even when the stimulus did not change, an increase in activity was observed prior to the transition from a perception of the ineffective stimulus to that of the effective one.

These results suggest a competition during the early stages of cortical processing between the two possible percepts. The activity of the cells in V1 and in V4 can be thought of as perceptual hypotheses, with the patterns across an ensemble of cells reflecting the strength of the different hypotheses. Interactions between these cells ensure that by the time the information reaches the IT lobe, one of these hypotheses has coalesced into a stable percept. Reflecting the properties of the real world, the brain is not fooled into believing two objects exist at the same place at the same time.

Random Dot Acuity

Before fleeing from Hungary to reach the US, Bela Julesz was a radar engineer with an interest in aerial reconnaissance. Spying from the air uses a clever trick of triangulation that is able to penetrate camouflaged objects on the ground. They photograph the ground once and then again after flying a few miles. The two pictures are then placed side-by-side in a stereo-viewer and scrutinized. Since each picture depicted an image from different vantage points, the viewer picked up the binocular depth cues in the pictures and easily saw through the camouflage.

Julesz was the first to consider using random-dot stereograms as a way of studying stereoscopic perception without the complications of monocular cues to depth. When viewed monocularly, each of the two stereo-targets appears as a random array of dots on a page arranged in similar sized squares. Each target by itself contains no information about the central square region in one being displaced laterally with respect to the same region in the other. This information only becomes evident when the two patterns are compared to each other, binocularly.

Observations using random-dot patterns have many important consequences for an understanding of binocular vision. When viewing random-dot stereograms at least, binocular fusion is achieved on a mosaic dot-by-dot basis and not by bringing together elaborated forms. Random-dot stereopsis suggests that the mechanism in the brain responsible for depth discrimination is independent of the eye of origin.

Why did natural selection equip primates with an ability to see shapes in stereo that neither eye could see individually? In other words, why did true cyclopean vision evolve instead of a simpler stereo system that could match up similar objects occurring at key locations within each retina?

A tentative explanation has to do with the fact that primates evolved in trees and had to negotiate a network of branches masked by dense foliage. The price of failing to discern discontinuities in the visual field would be a long drop to the forest floor below. Building a stereo "computer" into the binocular visual system would do the trick but only if the disparities were calculated over thousands of bits of visual texture, somewhat analogous to viewing a modern random-dot stereogram.

Since camouflage was discovered by the animal world ages before aerial surveillance technology, the earliest simians were able to see through the "hidden" insect's camouflage as it flattened its body against the tree bark. Such accurate Cyclopean vision provided the early primates with an effective countermeasure, revealing the prey just as aerial surveillance reveals hidden armored vehicles and weapon stores today.

So how does the so-called Cyclopean eye work?

David Marr, the late artificial intelligence researcher at MIT, was the first to describe vision as a means for animals to solve ill-posed problems of perception by carefully crafted assumptions about the world they inhabit. In other words, when parts of a puzzle cannot be solved one at a time, the puzzle-solver can keep in mind several informed *guesses* for each one. These are then compared for different parts of the puzzle to see which answers are mutually consistent with the final outcome.

Marr and Tomaso Poggio, a theoretical neuroscientist came up with a unique design for stereovision while viewing random-dot stereograms. The input units stand for points, such as the black and white squares of the stereogram. These feed into an array of units that represent all of the n x n possible matchups of a point in the left eye with some other point in the right.

When one of these units turns on, the network is guessing that there is a splotch at a particular depth in the visual field. Because the units are interconnected, the activation of one unit nudges the activation of its neighbors up and down the ocular columns. The activations reverberate throughout the cortex until it a global solution emerges that is consistent with the input. We experience the solution emerging but not the struggle of the processors to come up with a 3D percept.

Even though the Marr-Poggio model captures some essential features of how the brain computes stereovision, numerous experiments have shown that when subjects are introduced to "foreign" environments that tend to violate our everyday assumptions of how things work in this world, they are not as perturbed as what this model has us believe. This implies that the brain must be using additional information aids or concepts to help it figure out everyday issues or problems.

Nakayama and Shinsuke Shimojo created a random-dot stereogram whose depth information lay not in shifted dots but in dots that were visible in one eye's view and absent in the other's. Those dots lie at the corners of an imaginary square, with dots at the top, bottom right-hand corners present only in the right eye view and dots in the top, and bottom left corners only in the left eye's picture.

When subjects view the stereogram, they see a *floating* square defined by the four points. This shows that the brain indeed interprets features visible to only one eye as coming from an edge in visual space rather than just a series of unconnected dots. Nakayama and Barton Anderson, a psychologist, suggested that there are neurons that detect these occlusions, helping the stereo network extrapolate for the points that may be missing.

This finding does correlate well with numerous findings by other neuroscientists that imply that the brain does not like discontinuities in its visual field. For example, just like the visual cortex glosses over the so-called "blind spots" present in each eye, perceives a homogenous visual field, our "mind" fills in the perceptual gaps via experiential memory, and provides a coherent rationale of objects out there in 3D space.

Optical Illusions

How can the visual system compute the most probable 3D state of the world from the 2D input it receives from each retina?

First, it searches through its memory banks for an object that has the greatest likelihood of producing those lines or sketch based on the Occam's razor principle of parsimony, and

Second, it computes the probability of that particular object fitting the *context* of that visual scene (the proverbial zebra in the backyard scenario)

For example, a set of parallel lines are seldom an accident, for non-parallel lines in the world rarely project almost parallel lines in an image. Many laws in the natural world give it nice, analyzable shapes. Motion, tension and gravity make straight lines. Gravity makes right angles. Cohesion makes smooth contours.

However, vision is not a Cartesian theater designed by our awareness. We experience only the scene unfolding directly in front our eyes, the rest of it appears as a vague, peripheral smear of an ethereal existence. Our eyes flit from spot to spot several times a second forming an etch-n-sketch like image of the surroundings. We see in perspective. We are aware from experience that moving objects loom, shrink in size and foreshorten.

Ambient light also influences a lot of the visual field and certain built-in laws of constancy guide the visual cortex in arriving at appropriate rationales for what it is seeing. Since we are used to seeing surfaces rather than volumes, we have an almost palpable sense of surfaces and the boundaries between them. Some of the most famous illusions in optometry stem from the brain's unflagging struggle to carve the visual scene into surfaces and to decide where they would be likely to fit in the real world scenario.

For example, take the Kanisza triangle or the Rubin face profiles/vase illusions. The reason the viewer has such a hard time deciding between what is seen and what is actually there is because the brain knows intuitively that the picture is flat or 2D but is simulating 3D objects.

So what does the brain end up doing?

Marr, with tongue-in-cheek I am sure, chose to call it a $2^{1/}{}_2$D sketch while other researchers call it a visible-surface representation.

The information in this modified 2D array is specified in a retinal frame of reference, if you will, which simulates a coordinate system centered on the viewer. There are a series of reciprocal reference frames like the vestibular system, cerebellum and basal ganglia or the superior colliculus that compensate for movements of the head and body. They provide each bit of surface in the visual field a fixed address relative to the field, which stays the same as the body or eyes move.

Irv Biederman, a psychologist, has fleshed out Marr's ideas by invoking an inventory (24) of simple geometric forms called *geons*, which tend to be combinatorial. His theory suggests that at the highest levels of perception, the mind sees objects and parts as *idealized* geometric solids. These *geons* are not good for everything for many natural objects such as mountains and trees have complex fractal shapes.

In a highly social species like ours, or even the great apes taken together, face recognition and being able to "read" facial expressions is very important. Some studies suggest that face recognition may even use distinct parts of the brain. One famous set of experiments pointed to *mental rotation* of the object in view as central to successfully solving the dilemma such face or object recognition tasks pose to our brain.

Cooper and Shepard demonstrated that the brain rotates objects in mental space in order to decide its handedness, right or left or to figure out if it is a mirror image of the viewed object. Mental imagery drives our thinking about objects in space but we do not use such imagery to rearrange furniture or figure out where a person is sitting in a huge mansion. Many creative people claim to see the solution to a problem by visualizing it in an image.

For example, Crick and Watson mentally rotated models of what was to become the double helix; Einstein imagined what it would be like to ride on a beam of light. Painters and sculptors try out various ideas in their minds and novelists devise scenes and criminal plots in their mind's eye before putting it down on paper. Images drive the emotions as well as the intellect.

However, what is a mental image? Brain scientists call it a topographically organized cortical map i.e. a patch of cortex in which each neuron element responds to contours in a specific portion of the visual field. The primate brain has at least fifteen of these maps and truly, they are pictures in the head. As explained in previous sections, ambient space out there is represented by a topographical or contour map of the visual terrain.

The brain is also geared to interpret or integrate information flowing down from the limbic system with its memory stores into these mental images. Imagery can affect perception in gross ways too. Mental images of lines make it easier to judge alignment and can even induce visual illusions.

Perception

A central hypothesis in visual perception is that visual information is distributed across distinct subsystems. In this view, perception is analytic. The early processes are devoted to analyzing attributes of a stimulus: Some processes represent shape, while others mediate color and provide information about the dynamics or movement in the visual scene.

In some ways, this may sound almost counterintuitive for our perception of the things out there come across as a unified whole rather than a compilation of visual fragments. Nonetheless, as we shall see later on, converging evidence from various branches of cognitive neuroscience do provide compelling support for the idea that perception operates in an analytic manner.

Indeed, the feature-extraction hypothesis is one of the best examples of how cognitive optometry can provide complementary evidence of the central role played by the visual system in the complex process of cognitive perception. Although each visual area provides a map of external space, the maps differ with regard to the type of information they represent. For instance, neurons in some areas are highly sensitive to color variation. In other areas, the neurons may be movement sensitive but color insensitive.

By this hypothesis, neurons within this area not only code for where an object is located in visual space but also provide information about the object's salient attributes. Visual perception is, in other words, a divide-and-rule strategy. Rather than each visual area representing all attributes of an object, each provides its own limited analysis.

Image processing is distributed and specialized. As we advance through the visual system, different regions elaborate on the initial information gathered by the retina and begin to integrate it to form coherent, recognizable percepts. Extensive physiological evidence supports the specialization hypothesis.

For example, single-cell recordings in the M pathway show that these neurons are not specific in terms of the color of the stimulus. These cells extending from the magnocellular layer of the LGN through 4b and V2 respond similarly whether the colored circle is green or red but very specific to the direction of its motion.

Does visual imagery share space with vision in the brain? Numerous PET scans of subjects show that mental images do tend to be laid out across the visual cortical surface as a sort of crude depiction of the visual field. Interestingly, visual images though they share brain areas with perception are somehow different from the real display. Donald Symons asserts that reactivating a visual experience may well have benefits but it also may confuse imagination with reality.

That may be why within moments of awakening from a dream, our memory for its plot is wiped out, presumably to avoid contaminating autobiographical memory with bizarre confabulations. Similarly, our voluntary, waking mental images might be hobbled to keep them from becoming hallucinations or false memories.

Imagery is a wonderful faculty but we must not be carried away with the idea of pictures in the head. There is no such thing. We cannot reconstruct an image of an entire environment in our heads. We create fragments and collages in our heads. We recall glimpses of parts arrange them in a mental tableau and then sift through the fragments to refresh each one when it begins to fade.

In addition, visual memories are not accurate pictures of whole objects but a sort of caricature or cartoon depiction of the real thing. They cannot serve as adequate models or concepts to cognition or even perception. How can a concrete image represent an abstract concept? For example, how can one conceptualize an American or the idea of freedom or even what constitutes a human being?

Pictures are by definition ambiguous artifacts whereas thoughts cannot be. An image can be worth a thousand words but that is not necessarily such a good thing. At some point between gazing and thinking, images must give way to ideas and perception. Perception is found to be intimately interwoven with memory. Object recognition is more than linking features to form a coherent whole. That "big picture" triggers memories.

Are there separate representational systems for different types of information such as objects and faces? Do the sensory modalities have their own memory systems? Or, do they access a modality-independent knowledge base?

At an even more fundamental level, perception and recognition do not appear to be unitary phenomena but are manifest in many guises. As seen earlier, the pathways carrying visual information from the retina to the first few synapses in the cortex clearly segregate into multiple processing streams.

Early on there is partitioning into the M and P pathways followed by differential projection of the latter to blob and inter-blob zones in V1. But, once past the lower cortical regions, convergence and divergence become the anatomical rules leading to the so-called dorsal (where) pathway of the parietal lobe and the ventral (what) route of the temporal lobe. The neurons in both lobes have large receptive fields.

Neurons in the parietal lobe, however, have an interesting property in that they can respond in a non-selective way (react to both focal and ambient stimuli) in central and peripheral regions of the visual field. The temporal lobe neurons are activated by stimuli that fall within the left or right visual field but always encompassing the fovea. This disproportionate representation of central vision appears to be ideal for a system devoted to object recognition.

Cells within the visual areas of the temporal lobe have a diverse pattern of selectivity. One study employed a wide range of stimuli. Some were simple, involving edges or bars at orientations that varied in color or brightness. Others were complex and included photographs or 3D models of objects like a human head, hand, apple, flower and snake.

Of the 151 cells sampled, 110 consistently responded to at least one of the stimuli. A large minority (41%) acted similar to parietal neurons i.e. they were activated by any of the stimuli and their firing rates were similar across the set of stimuli. The remaining 59% exhibited some selectivity and responded more vigorously when viewing complex stimuli.

Recording from a cell located in the inferior temporal (IT) cortex displayed pronounced activity when viewing a model of the human hand. The activity was high regardless of the hand's orientation and was only slightly reduced when the hand model was considerably shrunk down.

To summarize, the what-where or what-how dichotomy offers a functional account of two computational goals for higher visual processing. This distinction is best viewed as a heuristic one rather than reflecting an absolute distinction. The dorsal and ventral pathways are not isolated from each other but communicate extensively. Processing within the parietal lobe, the termination of the "where" pathway serves many purposes.

It is known to play a critical role in selective attention and the enhancement of processing at some locations instead of others. Moreover, spatial information can also be useful for resolving "what" problems. For instance, depth cues help to segregate a complex scene into its component objects.

Object Recognition

Object recognition depends primarily on the analysis of the form of a visual stimulus, although cues such as color, texture and motion certainly contribute to normal perception. To account for shape-based recognition, two things need to be considered. The first has to do with shape encoding i.e. how is the shape internally represented. What salient features enable us to recognize differences between a triangle and a square or a monkey and a person?

The second center on how shape is processed when the perceiver's viewing position is rarely constant. We can recognize shapes from a wide array of positions and orientations since our recognition system is not hampered by scale changes in the retinal image as we move closer to or further away from an object.

A central debate in object recognition has to do with defining the frame of reference where recognition occurs. Two general approaches have been proposed: view-dependent and view-invariant recognition.

In view-dependent theories, perception is assumed to depend on recognizing an object from a specific viewpoint. They posit that we have a plethora of specific representations of varied objects in our memory bank. The viewer simply comes up with the closest appropriate match by visually rotating the object in mental space. The time needed to decide if two objects are similar or different increases as the viewpoints diverge.

In the view-invariant approach, object recognition does not occur by simply analyzing the stimulus information. Sensory input defines its basic properties and recognition may depend on an inferential process based on a few salient features.

Sensory information can change from one viewpoint to another. Nonetheless, the external world has certain basic architectural details that the visual system exploits during perception. The various "theories" of object recognition have emphasized the significance of such invariant properties with which we are able to infer our surroundings.

Ensemble Coding

The finding that neurons of the IT region of the temporal lobe selectively respond to complex stimuli agrees with the hierarchical theories of object perception. According to the Ensemble theory, V1 neurons code elementary features such as line orientation and color of the various objects in the visual field. Their outputs are then combined to form detectors sensitive to higher-order features such as corners, edges or intersections, an idea consistent with the findings of Hubel and Wiesel.

The process of reconstructing the outer scene progresses through each successive stage coding for combinations that are more complex until the collated information arrives at the IT. The neurons here are activated by specific shapes like hands or faces. This type of neuron has been called a *gnostic* unit, referring to the idea that they can signal the presence of a *known* stimulus - an object, place, animal or person that has been encountered by the observer in the past.

These so-called *gnostic* cells are representational elements that are infrequently active and so carry a lot of information when they do fire. Their firing corresponds to a complex feature i.e. mother's face/profile/ voice/ smell etc. in the sensory input. Thus, a small number of them can represent an entire scene and they can classify or categorize specific areas of the field in sensible ways.

With this population or ensemble hypothesis, recognition is not due to one unit but to collective activation. The ensemble theories readily account for why we tend to confuse one visually similar object or person with another. Losing some of these Gnostic cells might also degrade our ability to recognize an object.

Interestingly, it was discovered that the selectivity of these neurons is usually relative rather than absolute. They prefer certain stimuli to others but can also be "faked" into firing by ambiguous signals that may be visually similar.

Are human or animal faces special? Is there such a thing as a "Grandma" cell?

Some scientists assert that face perception may not be mediated by the same processing mechanisms as the ones for object recognition. One argument in favor of this hypothesis is based on primate and human evolution. The reasoning goes something like this: When we meet other individuals, we usually scrutinize their faces rather than the rest of the body, a behavior that is not newly acquired by humans but which has a long-standing history.

The tendency to focus on faces is found across most cultures around the globe and the study of facial expressions provide the most salient clues to the person's moods or emotional state.

Two decades of research confirmed that cells in two distinct regions of the temporal lobe are preferentially activated by faces; one in the superior temporal sulcus and the other in the inferior temporal gyrus. Numerous imaging studies have also confirmed engagement of the fusiform gyrus during a range of face perception tasks. Indeed, this region has come to be referred to as the fusiform face area (FFA) in literature.

However, even in the right hemisphere of the brain, the FFA does not appear to be exclusively activated by faces. Tasks requiring judgments about dogs or trees also produce activation in the FFA over baseline but to a lesser extent than actual faces. Thus, even though face perception appears to utilize distinct physical processing systems, we must keep in mind the problems with *single* dissociations as in the so-called "grandma" cell.

As the numerous studies point out, patients who have a selective disorder in face perception but have little problem with recognizing objects, does not imply a specialized processor mechanism for just faces. Perhaps the tests that assess face perception are more sensitive to the effects of brain damage than the ones evaluating objects.

When we consider the kind of tasks typically involved in assessing faces as opposed to objects, the patient has to decide between two faces (same category) versus a broad range of objects (different categories). Thus, face perception tasks involve within-category discrimination whereas object perception tasks involve between-category ones.

The goals-oriented aspects of perception that we use vision to guide our movements, to manipulate tools or to recognize faces underscore the selective aspects of cognition. Humans, and possibly some of the great apes are not passive processors of information. We can select from the dazzling array of neural impulses impinging upon our senses at any one time. Depending on our goals, the relative importance of various sources of information constantly changes.

Section 3

An Overview of Cognition

Animal 'Minds'

Most of us love our pets and cannot understand how people, especially well educated ones, still labor under the delusion that "animals are Cartesian machines and it is the availability of language that confers on us, first, the ability to be self-conscious and second the ability to feel". According to Macphail, there is no convincing evidence for consciousness in other species. They are not just devoid of speech and self-awareness but feelings too.

On the other hand, Baars argues that there are no fundamental biological differences that could justify denying subjectivity to other species for the known correlates of consciousness are phylogenetically ancient, going back to at least the early mammals.

From the observer's point of view, vision feels like an automatic process that helps map out the external, physical reality into the inner, mental universe. However, a few moments of introspection reveal that the relationship between these two worlds is far more complex. Experiences are not simply 'given', as some empiricists have asserted. Rather, your 'mind', implicitly or explicitly, selects the few nuggets of information that are of current relevance from the vast flood of data streaming in from the sensory periphery.

The prefrontal cortex is incapable of processing all this information. It deals with this information overload by *selectively attending* to a miniscule portion of it, neglecting most of the rest. By selectively attending to particular events or things out there, you choose to experience just one of the innumerable worlds out there clamoring for attention. What you are conscious of is usually what you attend to. Indeed, a venerable tradition in psychology equates consciousness of an object or event with attending to it.

However, it is important not to conflate these two notions. Attention and cognition are distinct processes and their relationship may be more intricate than conventionally envisioned. Some type of attentional selection is probably necessary but may not be sufficient for cognitive perception. When attending to something, the rest of the scene outside your 'focus' still goes on. Even when 'spacing-out' while driving or thinking, one does remain conscious of the gist of the scene in front of you.

Change blindness, where the observer fails to detect a large change between two otherwise identical images, inattentional blindness in which the magician performs obvious sleight-of-hand tricks right under one's nose are just two instances where some type of attentional selection or deficits occur.

Analogous to *ambient* vision, where any movement out in the peripheral field instantly captures the gazer's interest and compels foveation of the object, neuronal representation for *gist* perception mediates the rich sense of seeing or in this case, attending, to everything.

Neural Substrates of Attention

Attention is notoriously difficult to pin down precisely. Within the visual domain, with which I deal with on a constant basis, a long-standing metaphor for selective attention is that of a stage spotlight. Only the items illuminated by it are amenable for further processing and scrutiny. Neuronal selection mechanisms prevent information overload by letting only a fraction of all sensory data pass into awareness.

The process of activating the RAS can be visualized as the *'dimmer-switch'* on the spotlight. One can go from deep sleep to full intensity in seconds, with the proper training but as most of us notice on weekends, it may take a good fifteen to twenty minutes to ramp-up.

In keeping with this *'dimmer*-switch' concept of attention, it begins with the various stages of sleep at the low end of the rheostat when the entire CNS plods along in 'idle' mode. As the brainstem and thalamus come on-line, one gradually becomes 'aware' of the surroundings. The RAS then kicks it up another notch by recruiting the cerebral cortex. Now one goes through a gradual process of 'arousal'. You begin to show good 'orientation' as to time and place and are now considered fully alert and 'conscious'.

Depending upon the situation and ambient conditions, one can sustain this level of activity all day or, when duty calls, ramp it up to a state of vigilant alertness. When the *sympathetic* division of the autonomic nervous system is engaged, the 'fight-or- flight' mode is brought into place and the human acquires focused attention.

Electrophysiological studies of monkey and human brains reveal that focal attention can modulate responses throughout the cerebral cortex, including V1, V2, V4, MT, parietal and IT areas of the dorsal and ventral "streams", the premotor and prefrontal regions and the thalamus. Depending on context, attention may influence all levels of the cortical hierarchy beyond the retina.

The cellular manifestation of attention can be understood as helping one budding coalition establish dominance over other nascent coalitions. Little interference is expected as long as the relevant neuronal networks do not overlap when heading towards the inferior temporal (IT) cortex. These items are the ones the subject is aware of in the visual field under scrutiny.

Human electrophysiological and neuromagnetic recordings suggest the concept of early selection and extend it with evidence on the neural stages of perceptual processing that are likely involved. The general model supported by these data is that incoming sensory signals can be altered within the sensory-specific cortex when stimuli having relevant physical features are encountered.

The earliest form of this selection can be defined by location in auditory and visual systems. The implication of this data is that descending projections from attentional control systems affect the excitability of cortical neurons coding the features of the stimuli to be attended or ignored. The data also informs us about the sites (cortical vs. subcortical, sensory cortex vs. association areas etc.), where attentional effects are manifest during perceptual processing.

However, as vision scientists, we also want to know precisely which brain structures are being modulated as well as what systems and circuits are involved in the voluntary and reflexive control of these perceptual modulations. The modern methods of neuro-imaging of attentional control networks provide us with this data.

In addition to determining the activation of sensory-specific cortical areas, PET and fMRI studies of selective attention have revealed attention-related activity in several other brain areas: the pulvinar nucleus of the thalamus, the basal ganglia, the insular cortex, the frontal cortex, the anterior cingulate nucleus, the posterior parietal cortex and parts of the temporal lobe.

Some regions (frontal cortex, parietal cortex and pulvinar) are implicated in directing attention or when attention is switched to another target voluntarily (visual search task). These findings suggest that shifts of attention during such visual searches are subserved by the same neuronal machinery as the voluntary movements in response to various binocular cues.

If there are attentional modulations of the primary cortex, could they reflect earlier gating in the thalamus or even in the retina?

Unlike the cochlea, no neural projections to the human retinas can serve as a substrate for modulating retinal activity. However, in monkeys and other primates massive neuronal projections extend from the visual cortex back to the thalamus. These synapse in the *reticular* nucleus or more specifically in vision, on the *perigeniculate* nucleus (surrounding the LGN).

Another major subcortical structure that has been implicated in attentional processes as mentioned briefly above, is the pulvinar nucleus of the thalamus. We know that the pulvinar is activated during attentional filtering tasks. It has visually responsive neurons that show color, motion and orientation selectivity. In addition, it has subdivisions containing retinotopic maps of the visual field and interconnections with frontal, parietal, occipital and temporal cortical areas.

Single-cell recordings in awake *macaques* have demonstrated longer response latencies in neurons of the dorso-medial region of the lateral pulvinar (Pdm), than in other regions of the pulvinar. In addition, responses in these neurons are enhanced when the stimulus either is the target of a saccade or is attended without any eye movements. The bottom line is that the parietal cortex and subcortical structures like the pulvinar are key nuclei for orienting attention to relevant locations in the visual field.

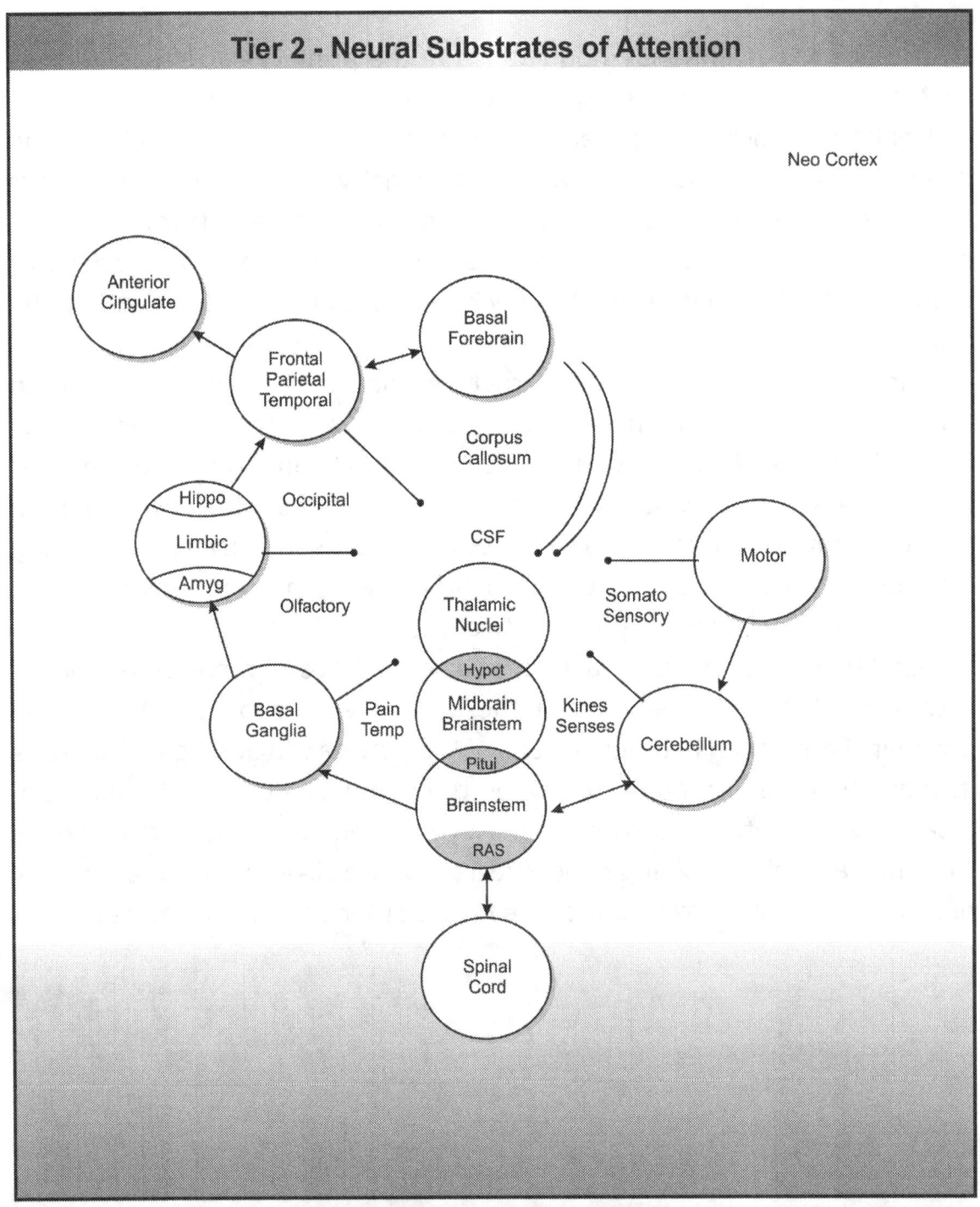

Neural Substrates of Attention:

A Diagrammatic representation

Selective Attention & Orienting

What we choose to attend to and what grabs our attention can dominate our experience. Precisely what neuronal mechanisms are involved when we concentrate our attention on external events or when they capture our awareness is one of the most intriguing issues in cognitive neuroscience. Consider the following question: Do you selectively decide to attend to things or to regions of space or both?

Spatial selective attention occurs in part via the modulation of sensory processes in the visual cortex. These effects happen primarily in extra-striate cortical areas but may also involve mechanisms in the striate. We can be certain that attention is acting on visual cortical processing for several reasons: first, the early P1 spatial attention effect has properties indicative of a visual sensory stage of processing.

Second, its latency (70 msec) is consistent with neuronal firing latencies in early extra-striate areas, as we know from research in monkeys. Finally, functional neuro-imaging performed in these paradigms localized attentional modulations of sensory processing to regions of extra-striate cortex as described below.

Attentional phenomena are diverse and entail many brain computations at various levels in the hierarchy of perception. The systems for mediating attention include the parietal lobe, temporal and frontal cortices and several subcortical structures. The result in visual processing, for example, is that we observe modulations in the electrical activity of neurons as they analyze and encode perceptual information.

Back in the 1950s, a British psychologist examined the so-called Cocktail Party effect, which delves into how people can focus on a single conversation in the noisy, confusing environment of a cocktail party. He found that selective auditory attention is the way to achieve your goal i.e. tune in on the interesting conversations while tuning out boring ones.

A key issue raised by the cocktail party experiments and the ensuing "gating" model of selective attention had to do with the stage(s) of stimulus processing where incoming signals can be selected or rejected by internal attentional processes. This is known as the "early-versus-late selection" idea in which cognitive psychologists asked about the extent of processing that supposedly ignored signals might actually attain.

In other words, if the subject is unaware of ignored conversations, perhaps s/he simply closed the "gate" on irrelevant inputs before they reached conscious awareness. One aspect of the early-versus-late selection debate is the concept of *limited capacity*, an idea that naturally flows from the observation that human performance suffers when overloaded by multiple inputs.

The early-and-late selection views assume that the human or animal information systems cannot simultaneously process multiple inputs if there is a high information load, so the system must make hard "decisions" about which task to tackle next.

Now, a processing "bottleneck" occurs where all inputs cannot gain access to or pass that stage of processing. This is thought to happen at key way stations during information processing, the presumption being that the cognitive system evolved selection mechanisms to "gate" information flow by establishing priorities.

Neuroscientists no longer wonder whether early or late selection is the key mechanism for selective attention because both are equally relevant. The fascinating fact is that physical stimuli that impinge on the retina may not be expressed in our conscious awareness, either in real time or later on via an imagery of our recollections.

Adaptation and the Brain

Evolutionists researching human behavior think that the modern human brain was adapted to deal with the world of the Pleistocene epoch, about 100,000 years ago. Therefore, when we think about the functions of the modern brain and what it does and does not do well, we should take into account what the early hunter-gatherers had to cope with.

Various studies of decision-making capacities in humans, argue that the mechanisms for decision- making evolved in a particular social context when humans lived for the most part in small groups. There may well be differences in how we make decisions in different social contexts, some tending to appear more irrational than others do. According to evolutionary thinking, these special capacities grow from separate and individual adaptations.

The cognitive system that evolved is thus not a 'unified' system that can work by applying specially crafted solutions to unique individual problems. The adaptations built into our brains are the neural networks, which set us apart from the rest of our great ape cousins. For example, the brainstem, which is the oldest part of the brain (400 million years ago) still, manages to retain, even to this day, many of the anatomical and functional characteristics. This is where we will begin our search for the initial birth of 'true' human consciousness.

The brainstem is literally the *stalk* of the brain, through which pass all the nerve fibers relaying signals of afferent input and efferent output between the spinal cord and the higher brain centers. It consists of the medulla, the pons and the mesencephalon or mid-brain. A continuous, fluid-filled cavity, part of the brain's ventricular system, stretches throughout the brainstem.

Nazir Brelvi, OD

It has two dilated parts: the 4th ventricle is at the level of the Medulla and Pons, whereas the 3rd ventricle lies in the diencephalon.

Examination of its internal structure shows that it is more diverse than the spinal cord. The gray matter is subdivided into several regions or nuclei that mediate common tasks, separated by wispy strands of white matter. It contains the cell bodies of neurons whose axons go out to the periphery to innervate the muscles and glands of the head region. It gives rise to 10 of the 12 pairs of the cranial nerves. The brainstem also receives many afferent fibers from the head and visceral cavities.

In a series of landmark studies in the late 1940's, Moruzzi and Magoun demonstrated that running through the entire brainstem is a core of 'diffuse' nervous tissue, called the Reticular Formation (RF). It controls the level of arousal or wakefulness in animals. In reality, the RF is not one homogeneous structure but rather a conglomerate of cell groups, which comprise of a vast number of small, multi-branched neurons.

It was noticed that *direct* electrical stimulation of this multi-faceted structure via microelectrodes, seemed to 'awaken' the forebrain. The EEG changed abruptly from the slow, high amplitude, synchronized waveforms characteristic of deep sleep to the fast, low amplitude, desynchronized activity typically found in the awakened animal.

This notion of a 'monolithic' activating system has given way currently to the realization that 40 or more highly heterogeneous nuclei with novel cell structures are housed within the brainstem. The basic cyto-architecture of each cellular cluster is extremely 'amorphous' in stark contrast to the linear, layered organization of the cerebral cortex. The cells in these clusters manufacture, store and release numerous neuro-modulating agents such as acetylcholine, serotonin, dopamine, norepinephrine, histamine etc.

These receive and integrate information from many afferent pathways as well as from many cortical areas of both cerebral hemispheres. Essentially, the RF attends to tasks involving complex behaviors, which include the control of body posture, orientation of the head and body toward external stimuli, control of eye movements etc.

A considerable number of spinoreticular fibers project to widespread regions of the brainstem reticular formation. These fibers are predominantly uncrossed and terminate chiefly upon cells of the nucleus gigantocellularis of the medulla. The spinoreticular fibers passing to pontine levels are distributed bilaterally in the pontine reticular nuclei.

A small number of spinoreticular fibers reach the midbrain reticular formation. Functionally, the spinoreticular fibers play a significant role in behavioral awareness and in the modulation of electrocortical activities.

Two relatively large regions of the brainstem RF give rise to fibers that descend to spinal levels. One is in the pontine tegmentum, while the other lies in the medulla.

Experimental studies indicate that stimulation of the brainstem RF can:

(1)   Facilitate and inhibit voluntary movement, cortically induced movement and reflex activity,

(2)   Influence muscle tone, probably via the gamma system,

(3)   Affect phasic activities associated with respiration,

(4)   Exert pressor and depressor effects upon the circulatory system, and

(5)   Exert facilitating and inhibiting influences upon the central transmission of sensory impulses.

Areas of the medullary RF from which the medullary reticulospinal tract arises correspond to regions from which inspiratory, inhibitory and depressor effects are elicited. The facilitory, expiratory and pressor effects are obtained from regions rostral to the medulla.

The brainstem RF also receives inputs via cortico-reticular projections from widespread areas of the cerebral cortex, although the greatest numbers originate from the 'motor area'. The regions of termination correspond to those that give rise to the reticulo-spinal tracts. Thus, the synaptic linkages of cortico-reticular and reticulo-spinal fibers form a pathway from the cortex to spinal levels. There is no evidence of a somatotopic arrangement within this system.

Finally, most of the autonomic pathways originating in or relayed via hypothalamic neurons, project to the autonomic centers in the brainstem tegmentum, which relay the impulses to the various spinal neurons.

Locus Coeruleus and the Raphe Nuclei

Near the central gray of the upper part of the 4th ventricle and under its floor, lies an irregular but compact 'mass' of approximately 15,000 deeply pigmented neurons known as the Locus Coeruleus (LC). It appears to be present in all mammalian species. Fluorescein studies have revealed that the cells of this region contain catecholamines, practically all of which are norepinephrine.

Such adrenergic pathways, originating from the LC ascend to diencephalic levels, distributing widely in the cerebral cortex, the hypothalamus, the basal ganglia and the hippocampal formation, some even terminating in the cerebellum. Their organization appears to influence neural activity simultaneously in broad cortical regions of the brain. These neurons respond preferentially to novel 'exciting' stimuli and play an important role in mediating 'arousal', wakefulness and the control of sleep.

The Raphe nuclei form a narrow strip of neurons running along the midline of the medulla, pons and midbrain. They contain cell groups that technically belong to the Reticular Formation (RF), but appear to serve distinctive functions. Together, the raphe nuclei receive afferents from the cerebral cortex, hypothalamus and the RF while the efferents travel south to the spinal cord and north towards the cerebellum, PAG, hypothalamus, thalamus, hippocampus, amygdala, regions of the striatum and several septal nuclei.

Histofluorescent studies demonstrate that these cells contain stores of serotonin and other monoamines. Both serotonin and norepinephrine-containing neurons in the RF play active roles in the mechanisms that control sleep states, moods and emotions.

136

Inhibition of serotonin synthesis or the total destruction of the serotonin-containing neurons in the Raphe system leads to total insomnia. Serotonin appears to be involved in the neural mechanism related to so-called slow wave sleep. In addition, serotonin seems to modulate the neurons of the locus coeruleus region, which trigger REM or paradoxical sleep.

A final peculiarity of the raphe nuclei is that they send fibers to the ependymal cells, which line the inner aspects of the brain ventricles. Their function remains unknown but the presence of serotonin raises speculation of homeostatic control mechanisms.

The Hierarchy of Cognition

Visualize cognition as a complex *pinball* game being played in 3D, with the brain as the actual machine and a series of silver balls representing multiple thought impulses being launched into it. Some of the balls will hug the sideboard and fall back into the retrieval bin at the base while others will do various circuits around the machine. One or two of these balls will end up lighting up the scoreboard with all the bells and whistles. These "thoughts" are the ones you will become "conscious" of and pay attention to.

Numerous electro-physiological experiments in both macaques and humans reveal that focal attention can modulate responses throughout the V1, V2, V4, MT, the parietal and IT areas of the dorsal and ventral pathways, the thalamus and some specific structures of the premotor and prefrontal cortex. The V4 and posterior IT (PIT) are key players in the attentional modulation of perceptual tasks. Without these regions, animals can still discriminate an isolated target but not when embedded within a busy collage.

Depending on the ambient conditions, attention may act at practically all levels beyond the retina: from the LGN right into the primary visual cortex. It heightens the *gain* of the sensory apparatus by not only affecting the firing rate of the neurons but also increasing their *spike coherency* (synchrony), thereby boosting their postsynaptic punch.

Basically, cognition can be regarded as *enhanced awareness*, if you will, wherein the animal is not only attending to the scene but also oriented towards it with certain intentionality. For example, a cat stalking a bird out in the meadow. It is focused intently on its task and even though not really interested in killing the bird for food, perfectly willing to bring it down. Here attention, mediated by the cat's reticular activating system (RAS) in conjunction with some other sensory modalities, is involved in *priming* the cat's brain for further action.

In other words, as its stalking progresses, the cat is on the alert for any eventuality. Cognition enters the scene when the status quo is disturbed i.e. the bird catches on and escapes or decides to attack the stalker. In either case, the cat now puts plan B in action: fight or run away. Now, the cat's entire brain is lit up. Not only is the predator's visual system (from the retina to the higher visual cortex) but the amygdala (fear), hippocampus (stored memories), basal ganglia and cerebellum (motor actions) and the rest of the cerebral hemispheres (IT, MT, premotor, prefrontal etc., etc.) are roped into the fray.

The cat is beginning to cognate, to think. However, its thinking is much unlike ours. Its brain is processing sensory information for action rather than perception. A classic study performed by two neurologists from the University of Durham in England makes this dichotomy clear. They discovered a multitude of visuo-motor systems, each controlling a specific behavior, such as eye movements, posture adjustment, hand gripping or pointing, foot placement and so on, yet none giving rise to conscious sensation.

These visuo-motor behaviors care about the here and now and do not need to access long-term memory systems well hidden away in the hippocampus. In fact, numerous psychophysical experiments show quite conclusively that enforcing a delay of 2-4 seconds between a brief visual input (via a tachistoscope) with a concomitant hand or eye movement taps into a *different* spatial map of the world in humans.

In the so-called lower animals, like the cat in the above-mentioned example, the path taken by the vision-for-action scenario is used to execute a near-instantaneous motor response. There is no reason to access the higher cortical regions mediating conscious perception or sentience as found in the primates and humans. In the predatory cats its all in the here and now. They get hungry, they kill and eat. Hunger satisfied, they rest and sleep.

In other words, the process of Cognition refers to the ability and capacity of an organism to attend or focus in on an evolving situation, in real time. It follows a standard course and usually runs for about 500 msecs. Within this half-a second, the creature has acquired, evaluated, understood and decided on a plan of action.

The so-called cognitive circuit encompasses the entire brain from the brainstem, thalamus, corpus callosum to the sensory cortices (parietal, temporal, occipital lobes), to the cingulate gyrus (various nuclei of the limbic system), prefrontal cortex and out through the premotor cortex, basal ganglia, thalamus, hypothalamus, pituitary, motor cortex, cerebellum, pons medulla and spinal cord.

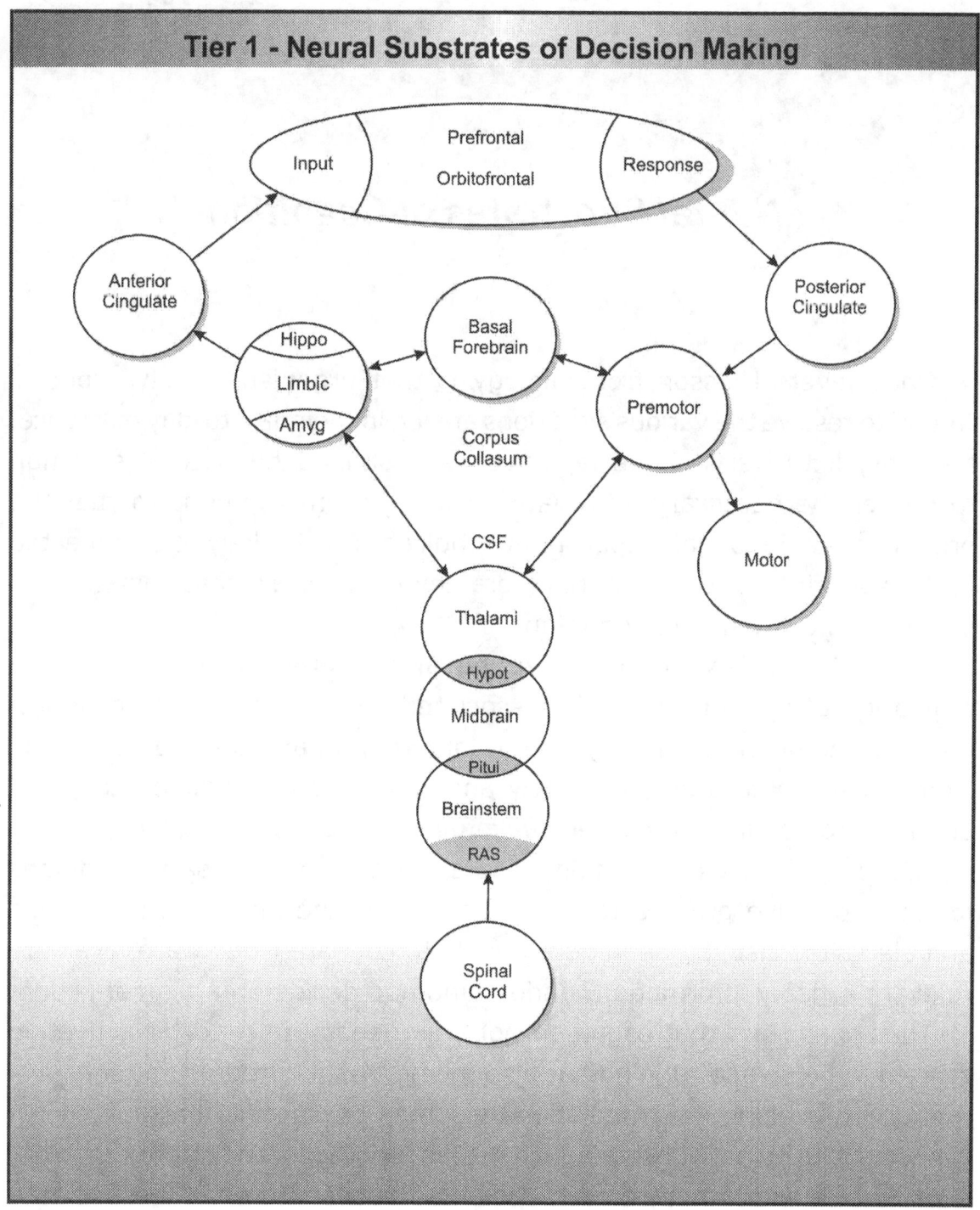

Neural Substrates of Decision Making

Neural Substrates of Cognition

One universal lesson from biology is that organisms evolve specific "tools" to resolve the various situations arising in their day-to-day existence. Neurons, like everything else, have been shaped by natural selection to gather the necessary information from the environment so that the organism is able to make appropriate choices. This is likely to be reflected in the specificity of the neuronal hierarchy of the brain that confers onto it the complex mantle of cognition.

The ability to experience anything at all depends on the ongoing regulation of the cortex and its associated structures by a collection of nuclei in the brainstem (RAS), the basal forebrain and the thalamus. The axons of these cells project widely and release acetylcholine (Ach) and other neuromodulators to affect wakefulness, arousal and sleep.

Collectively, these ascending fibers create the necessary conditions for any cognitive process to occur, because if the animal is not awake and alert, it is also, by definition, unable to cognate (be aware, evaluate relevant sensory information, understand and decide on a plan of action.

Thus it appears that cognition not only needs the reticular activating system to be up and running but also the neuronal output from regions of the forebrain along with mediation by some non-specific thalamic nuclei. (These nuclei do not subserve any one sensory modality but project to the superficial layers of many cortical regions. The best known of these are the intralaminar nuclei, which when lesioned seem to knock out all awareness in the individual with no tangible evidence of mental functioning.)

Since one of the principal functions of cognition is figuring out how to outwit the predator or fellow chimp with all that food, the individual

142

has to be able to formulate some kind of *action* plan. This suggests that the neural substrates are intimately linked to the planning and executive centers of the brain, localized, roughly speaking, in the prefrontal region of the brain.

Moreover, the two cerebral cortices are connected by the largest fiber system in the brain, the corpus callosum. In humans, this bundle of white matter includes more than 200 *million* axons. Many of the callosal projections link together homotopic areas (corresponding locations) in the two hemispheres but mainly in the association areas not in the primary cortices. The callosal fibers also project to heterotopic areas i.e. prefrontal to premotor but these tend to be less extensive than comparable projections within the same hemisphere.

The functional role of callosal projections remains unclear. Some researchers point out that in the visual association cortex, receptive fields can span both visual fields. Communication across the callosum enables information from both fields to contribute to the activity of these cells. Indeed, the callosal connections could play a role in synchronizing oscillatory activity in cortical neurons as an object passes through these receptive fields.

(Author's note: In neurological parlance, the connection between two cortical areas is said to be *ascending* if the axons predominately terminate in layer 4. This is particularly true if the cell bodies of the projection neurons that give rise to these axons are sited in the superficial layers 2 and 3.

A *descending* or feedback connection is one in which the axons avoid layer 4, targeting the upper layers instead (in particular, layer 1, the most superficial one) and on occasion, layer 6 (the deepest layer).

The cell bodies of the large pyramidal neurons that supply the feedback axons are usually found in deep layers.

The so-called *termination zone* of axons feeding back information from a higher to a lower level is wider than that of forward projecting neurons making excitatory synaptic contacts with a larger set of neurons.

Besides ascending and descending links, there are lateral connections too, which couple cortical areas at the same level in the hierarchy. Lateral connections can originate in all layers that project out of a cortical area i.e.

from all except layers 1 and 4, and can terminate throughout the width of the cortical column in the receiving area.

Yet despite the complexity of the linkages, not every area "talks" to every other one in the cortex. In fact, only about a third of all possible connections among areas have been reported so far.)

The twin thalami of each hemisphere are bordered medially by the 3rd ventricle, dorsally by the fornix and corpus callosum and laterally by the internal capsule, which is composed of projection fibers from the motor cortex to regions of the brainstem and spinal cord. It separates the thalamus from the basal ganglia. In some individuals, a short bridge of gray matter called the *massa intermedia* links the two thalami.

The thalamus has rightfully been referred to as the "gateway to the cortex" because with the exception of some olfactory inputs, all sensory modalities make synaptic relays in its various nuclei before continuing on to the primary cortical receiving areas. As seen in our discussion of the pulvinar and LGN earlier, the thalamic nuclei also receive inputs from and provide reciprocal feedback to the basal ganglia, cerebellum, neocortex and medial temporal lobe.

These descending cortico-thalamic projections terminate in a thin layer of cells that runs all along the margins of the thalamus. Neurons in this thalamic reticular nucleus form a lateral inhibitory network of cells that play an important role in the modulation of outputs projected by the specific thalamic subdivisions they overlay.

Below the thalamus is a small collection of nuclei and fiber tracts that lie on the floor of the 3rd ventricle known as the hypothalamus. It plays a central role in both the autonomic nervous system (ANS) and endocrine systems of the body, helping maintain internal balance or homeostasis. The hypothalamus is also involved in emotional processes and in the control of the pituitary gland that is attached to its base.

The hypothalamus not only receives inputs from the limbic cortex but also from the mesencephalic RF, amygdala and regions of the retina to modulate the circadian rhythms or light-dark cycles of the individual. Projections from the hypothalamus include a major one to the prefrontal cortex, amygdala and spinal cord and another to the pituitary. In addition to the direct neuronal projections, the hypothalamus also secretes several peptide hormones into the bloodstream that influence a wide range of behaviors farther afield.

The brainstem contains numerous groups of motor and sensory nuclei along with several ascending (sensory) and descending (motor) tracts. The organization becomes more complex as it proceeds from the spinal cord through the medulla, pons and midbrain to the diencephalon and cortex. This neural complexity reflects its underlying importance in mediating life-sustaining mechanisms such as respiration, heartbeats and even various states of consciousness like sleep and wakefulness.

The midbrain contains neurons that participate in visuomotor functions (e.g. superior colliculus, oculomotor n., trochlear n. etc.), visual reflexes (e.g. pretectal region), auditory relays (inferior colliculus) and the mesencephalic tegmental nuclei involved in fine motor coordination (Red nucleus). Much of the midbrain is occupied by the mesencephalic RF, which is a rostral continuation of the pontine and medullary RFs. Another major structure of the midbrain is the substantia nigra, a darkish collection of dopaminergic neurons that project to the caudate and putamen nuclei of the basal ganglia.

As described earlier, projection systems arising in the locus coeruleus, a midbrain nucleus, project widely to the cortex, uses norepinephrine as their main neurotransmitter. In a similar fashion, the raphe nuclei also project widely to the cortex but use serotonin as their main neurotransmitter. Finally, in addition to the projections of the substantia nigra noted above, the ventral tegmental region contains dopaminergic neurons that project throughout the cortex. Such biogenic amines and their projection systems are involved in a variety of modulatory functions in the brain and spinal cord.

The last areas of the brainstem to consider are the pons and medulla. Apart from a major portion of the RF, the pons consists of a vast system of cortical projections to regions of the brainstem, spinal cord and cerebellum, interspersed with several pontine tegmental nuclei located on the floor of the 4th ventricle. These nuclei mediate auditory and vestibular functions. Others relay sensory and motor impulses from the face and mouth while the visuomotor nuclei control some of the extraocular muscles of the eye.

The medulla has two prominent bilateral nuclear groups on the ventral surface (the gracile and cuneate nuclei) that serve as the primary relays for ascending somatosensory information entering the spinal cord and heading towards the thalamus and parietal lobes. The cortico-spinal projections form tight bundles (the pyramids) and *decussate* at the medulla in order to project to the contralateral side of the spinal cord.

At the rostral end of the medulla are the large nuclei of the olivary complex, part of the cortical-cerebellar motor system. These nuclei receive inputs from the cortex and red nucleus and project them to the cerebellum. Sensory nuclei that carry vestibular signals and some sensory inputs from the face, mouth, throat and abdomen lie here along with the motor nuclei that innervate the heart, muscles of the neck, tongue and throat.

Role of Basal Ganglia in Cognition& Learning

Patients who have had Parkinson's dss for a few years perform below normal on various tests of neuropsychological function. Given the anatomical links between the basal ganglia (BG) and the prefrontal cortex, researchers have explored how the motor problems observed in such patients might impinge on cognitive tasks. Known popularly as the Shifting hypothesis because the basal ganglia mediate the patient's shifting from one action to the next, it offers a unified framework for understanding BG function in both action and cognition.

BG monitor activation across wide regions of the cortex, allowing a shift between different actions and mental sets by removing an inhibitory influence in selected neurons. Recent studies demonstrate that the shifting operation is neither strictly motoric nor cognitive but rather a necessary link between mental set and action.

This shifting hypothesis may also hold the key to the BG's role in learning. Dopamine is known to play a critical role in the reward systems of the brain. It provides the animal with a neurochemical marker of the reinforcement contingencies that exist for different responses. In humans, it might mean recognizing that a demanding problem cannot be solved by conventional means.

One can hypothesize that within the BG, dopamine serves to bias the system to produce certain responses over others. It is released in the striatum following successful actions. A failure to shift may result in an absence of movement (as in Parkinson's dss) or the repetitive production of stereotyped movement patterns (as in OCD or Tourette's syndrome).

In either case, BG dysfunction makes it difficult to select new actions that arise when sensory input or internal goals change.

Learning & Memory

What is the relationship between learning and memory?

Learning is the process of acquiring new information, whereas memory refers to the persistence of learning in a state that can be revealed later. Learning then has an outcome and we refer to that as memory. In other words, learning happens when a memory is created or strengthened by repetition.

This need not involve a conscious attempt to learn. Learning can occur and performance can improve simply from more exposure to information or to a task. For example, we remember the details of a person's face better by seeing it more without having to try to consciously memorize facial features.

Learning and memory can be subdivided into major hypothetical stages: encoding, storage and retrieval. Encoding refers to the processing of incoming information to be stored. The encoding stage has two steps: acquisition and consolidation. Acquisition registers input in sensory buffers and sensory analysis stages, while consolidation creates a stronger representation over time.

Storage, the result of acquisition and consolidation, creates and maintains a permanent record. Finally, retrieval utilizes stored information to create a conscious representation or to execute a learned behavior like a motor act.

Memory theories include two main distinctions about how we learn and retain knowledge. The first is that memory can be defined by retention time. Thus, we have identified sensory memory, short-term/working memory and long-term memory. The second main concept involves the ideas that

Nazir Brelvi, OD

memories can be characterized by their content and that different types of information can be retained in partially or wholly distinct memory systems.

For example, we have identified several sub-types of long-term memory. The main distinction is the declarative versus non-declarative dichotomy. Knowledge is sometimes in the form of declarative memories, which are memories of events from our lives or even world knowledge that we have conscious access to and make declarations about.

Other forms of knowledge can be said to be non-declarative, which involves procedural knowledge (play a piano), perceptual priming, conditioned responses and non-associative learning. The information stored as non-declarative memory is typically out of reach of our conscious awareness.

The question that remains is whether these different memory systems are supported by different neural circuits and systems in the brain. If they were, we would have converging evidence for the idea that these qualitatively different forms of learning and memory are reflections of distinct memory mechanisms.

Cognitive theory and neuroscientific evidence reveal that memory is supported by multiple cognitive and neural systems. These systems support different aspects of memory and their distinctions in quality can be readily identified. Sensory registration, perceptual representation, working memory, procedural memory, semantic memory and episodic memory all represent systems or sub-systems for learning and memory. The brain structures that support various memory processes differ, depending on the type of information to be retained and how it is encoded or retrieved.

The biological memory system includes the medial temporal (MT) lobe, which forms and consolidates new episodic and perhaps semantic memories; the prefrontal cortex, which is involved in encoding and retrieval of information; the temporal cortex, which stores episodic and semantic knowledge; and the association sensory cortices for the effects of perceptual priming.

Other cortical and sub-cortical structures participate in learning skills and habits, especially those with implicit motor learning. The data from studies in human amnesic patients, in animals and in normal volunteers using electrophysiological and neuro-imaging methods permit us to elaborate on the cognitive model. The brain is not equipotent in the storage of information and although widespread brain areas cooperate in learning and memory, the individual structures form systems that support and enable rather specific memory processes.

At the cellular level, the variability in synaptic strengths between neural networks in the medial temporal (MT) lobe, neocortex and elsewhere are the most likely mechanisms for learning and memory.

Edelman and Tononi consider memory to be a *central* component of the brain mechanisms that mediates consciousness. They question the widespread assumption that memory involves the inscription and storage of information in some kind of coded form. They see it as being *nonrepresentational*, resulting from the *selective* matching that occurs between the ongoing, distributed neural activity and various signals from the world at large. The synaptic alterations that ensue affect the future responses of the individual brain to similar or different signals during recall.

Such a memory has properties that allow perception to alter recall and vice versa. It is robust, dynamic, associative and adaptive with an unlimited capacity. It is not strictly replicative like the one found in computers, which tends to be representational and follows a specified, predetermined code but creative since it generates 'information' by actual construction in real time.

In this view, there are hundreds, if not thousands of separate memory systems in the brain, which can range from all the perceptual systems in different modalities: vision, smell, touch, hearing etc., to ones that govern intended or actual movement, to the multi-variant language systems, which organize the complex sounds of human speech

Role of Emotions in Cognition

The belief that emotions are animal legacies from our ancestral apes, snarling and biting their way through conflicts, is a familiar depiction in pop ethology documentaries and the Discovery channel but quite untrue. Most parts of the human body did come from ancient mammals and before them ancient reptiles but the parts are heavily modified to fit human anatomy and physiology.

Emotional *repertoires* vary wildly among animals depending on species, gender and age. The common chimp often dwell in "gangs" in which belligerent males have been known to massacre rival bands, mount complex monkey hunts and indulge in frank cannibalism while the female sex have been observed to commit infanticide with impunity or snatch another's baby and rip it to shreds.

Their bonobo cousins, on the other hand, profess social alacrity, mount anyone around them sexually and go about living the *vida loca* till well into adulthood.

There is no question that moods dramatically affect human lives and behavior. Moods and emotions are also critical for survival and affect the way we perceive things out there. The systems work in tandem, integrated by many reciprocal connections. Most primates are not information-processing machines but rather motivated, emotional and social creatures. They are endowed with one of the most fundamental of human-like characteristics: the ability to feel emotions and express them.

Although there is considerable debate as to whether any single list is adequate to capture the vast nuances of emotional experience displayed in the world at large, most people would accept the idea that there are a finite number of basic, universal human emotions like happiness, sadness, fear, disgust, anger or surprise. These can be easily depicted via a series of facial expressions or reactions to events in the world that vary along a continuum.

One factor that differentiated emotion form other behaviors is that emotion alters not only our mental and neural states but also our physiological state. Emotional responses can bring about a number of bodily reactions because of activating the autonomic nervous system (ANS). For example, a late night jaunt through the alleyways of downtown Manhattan can speed up your heart, raise goose bumps or even induce some anxiety upon hearing quick footsteps behind you.

(Author's note: This idea that emotions alter our physiological state and that we can determine an emotional reaction by measuring our body's response is the basic principle behind the lie-detector test.)

However, is there a clear dividing line between emotion and cognition?

One of the more recent debates addressing this issue occurred between Robert Zajonc of Stanford and Richard Lazarus of UCal, Berkeley. Zajonc argued that *affective* judgments occur before and independently of cognition whereas Lazarus asserted that emotion could not occur without cognitive appraisal.

The primary issues in this debate hinged largely on how one defined cognition. Zajonc defined it as a slower mental transformation of sensory input or information processing. His studies were conducted to show dissociations between evaluation and awareness. For example, emotional stimuli were presented subliminally and so quickly, that subjects did not report, "seeing" them but seemed to influence how the subjects evaluated emotionally neutral stimuli that followed.

Lazarus defined cognition as including early evaluative perception as well as later stages of information processing. For example, if we experience signs of ANS arousal such as sweating, increased heart rate and blushing, our emotional response will depend on whether we are working out, having an interlude with a ravishing brunette or looking down from the glass floor of the CN Tower in Toronto.

In other words, the emotional response depends on the reason we believe we are experiencing the arousal. He believed that emotions were a subset of cognitive processes. One benefit of the recent work on the influence of emotions on cognitive processes is that by identifying some of the brain systems of emotion, we have shifted the debate to more neutral grounds. For instance we now know that some brain structures, like the amygdala, is specialized to process emotional stimuli and can respond very quickly and early in the processing of these stimuli.

These findings seem to be consistent with Zajonc's position that we have separate systems for the processing emotion. At the same time, the neural structures that are specialized for emotion can interact with and be influenced by neural systems known to mediate other cognitive behaviors. These results, however, suggest that emotion and cognition are interdependent, invoking Lazarus's proposal.

The Romantic Movement in philosophy, literature and art began about 200 years ago and since then the emotions and cognition (rational thought) have been assigned to different realms. In their view, emotions come from the body as hot irrational impulses compelling animal-like behavior while cognition seems to mediate civilized more human-like interactions.

The Romantics believe that emotions are the source of spontaneity, wisdom and creative genius and should be allowed free rein. Intelligence or cognitive perception, on the other hand, follows the interests of self and society by keeping the emotions in check.

Interestingly, Romanticism dominates contemporary American pop "culture" and is disseminated throughout the globe via formula films, inane psychobabble and sooth-saying charlatans of multimedia who are laughing all the way to their banks. Most Freudian psychologists tacitly accept the basic tenets of Romanticism in the form of the *id*, the *superego* and the diverse biological drives inherent in the human psyche even though they may implicitly disagree with its moral norms.

The modern infatuation with human emotions and consequent effects on behavior began with the so-called Triune brain theory initially proposed by Paul MacLean, a neuroscientist in the early 1970's. He took the Romantic doctrine and translated it into neuroscience by describing the human brain as an evolutionary *palimpsest* of three entities:

The *reptilian* brain as being responsible for primitive and selfish emotions that drive the four F's of feeding, fighting, fleeing and fornication.

Grafted onto it, was the limbic system or *primitive* mammalian brain, thought to mediate kinder, gentler social emotions like parenting.

Moreover, wrapped around these two was the *modern* mammalian brain or neocortex, which was believed to house the tumultuous emotional baggage of *archaic* humans dwelling in the Paleolithic epoch of yesteryears.

After an unbelievable run of nearly *four* decades, this theory was finally relegated to the recycle bin as neuroscientists realized that natural selection does not just heap layers of cortical matter willy-nilly. It tinkers and modifies the neural substrates of cognition and emotions to fit modern lifestyles.

The Limbic System: A Modern Approach

On the medial surface of the cerebral hemispheres on either side lies a large *arcuate* convolution formed primarily by the cingulate and parahippocampal gyri. Collectively known as the '*grande lobe limbique*', these surround the rostral brainstem, the inter-hemispheric commissures, the hippocampal formation and the dentate gyrus.

From a phylogenetic and cytoarchitectural point of view, the limbic lobe consists of the allocortex (hippocampal formation and dentate gyrus), the paleocortex (pyriform cortex of the anterior parahippocampal gyrus) and the mesocortex (cingulate gyrus). The striking feature of the limbic lobe is that it appears early in phylogenesis and possesses a certain constancy in gross and microscopic structure.

The designation of the limbic system stands for an even more extensive and inclusive term, used to include all of the limbic lobe and its associated subcortical nuclei i.e. the amygdaloid complex, the orbitofrontal cortex, the septal nuclei, hypothalamus, epithalamus and various thalamic nuclei. The medial tegmental region of the midbrain is also included since it contains both the ascending and descending pathways subserving the hippocampal formation and the amygdaloid nuclear complex.

Despite the heterogeneity and diffuse nature of the so-called limbic system, there are compelling observations that the structures comprising it are involved in neural circuitry that gives rise to a 'subcortical continuum'. It begins in the septal area and seems to extend to the paramedian zone through the preoptic region and then via the hypothalamus into the rostral mesencephalon.

The intimate relationship of the limbic lobe with the hypothalamus has led some neuroscientists to regard the limbic system as a whole to function as 'a visceral brain'. In humans, it seems to occupy a central position in mediating behavior and the complex world of emotions.

Over the years, the investigation of emotion has intensified. Researchers now acknowledge that emotion, especially in humans, is a multi-faceted behavior that is not amenable to a simple definition or mediation via a single neural circuit or cortical system. Studies of the cognitive neuroscience of emotion have invoked a number of brain regions with the orbitofrontal cortex and the amygdala emerging as prime suspects.

As we gain a greater understanding of the relative roles of these neural structures in emotional processing, it has become more apparent that we need to understand how these neural systems and others interact to produce normal and adaptive emotional responses.

For instance, most of the immediate focus on generating and comprehending the spoken words takes place in the prefrontal lobes within *milliseconds*, while their emotional content is mediated by the amygdala via the pituitary gland over the next few *minutes*. This apparent mismatch in 'processing' gives 'meaning' and context to the scene i.e. Qualia. The amygdala largely operates below conscious awareness and regulates autonomic behavior that we cannot directly control.

Perhaps the most important insight to come out of the growing understanding of our brain's chemistry is what the experts call 'mood congruity' i.e. the brain tends to record not only the specific details of the event but also our feelings about it. Our memory system tends to serve up recollections of past events that are themselves 'congruous' or similar in emotional content to your current mood. Our emotional state *skews* our sense of perspective by seeking out memories that match our current mind-set instead of a balanced, representative sample.

Emotions do not merely mark certain memories as being more important than others are. They also affect which details are recorded. Images that trigger strong emotional responses are recalled more readily than neutral ones. In addition, interestingly, so-called 'happy' images leave behind more of a generalized feeling of pleasantness while negative ones are recalled in excruciating detail.

We are also 'wired' to remember novelty and events that somehow deviate from expectation. In fact, we tend to *dwell* on events that take us by surprise. Researchers now believe that there is an entire neurochemical system devoted to the pursuit and recognition of new experiences and surprise, particularly ones pertaining to reward. It is regulated by Dopamine, one of the brain's 'reward' drugs.

If the pleasure factor of a certain event exceeds expectations than there is a spike in dopamine presence within the system, whereas disappointment causes a dramatic reduction. It is also believed that chronically low levels of dopamine play an important role in 'addictive' behaviors.

The last among the limbic structures we shall address are the hippocampus and adjoining regions of the temporal lobe, the dentate gyrus, the subiculum and the entorhinal area of the parahippocampal gyrus. Collectively these form the hippocampal formation (HF), which is precisely organized with several different cell types interconnecting in highly complex patterns.

Two aspects of these connections are central to understand its functional roles in mediating cognition: first, the extensive reciprocal connections with numerous cortical association areas and second, the direct and indirect links with other limbic structures (amygdala, cingulate gyrus and septal nuclei).

As for the neocortical connections, the hippocampus obviously processes large amounts of information. The parallel increase in its size during evolution furthermore indicates that its main functions are related to the neocortex. The quantitatively dominating afferent inputs to the dentate gyrus and the hippocampus arise in the entorhinal area. This area receives afferents from nearby association areas (the parahippocampal and perirhinal cortices) of the temporal lobe and integrates various kinds of sensory information from the cingulate gyrus, the insula and the prefrontal cortex.

The neurons of the dentate gyrus send their efferents to the hippocampus, whereas the hippocampal neurons project to the subiculum. From here, the fibers travel through the fornix to the mammillary nucleus and back to the entorhinal area. A large number of commissural fibers also connect the hippocampi of either lobe indicating a close cooperation between them.

The main flow of information from the hippocampus via the subiculum is directed toward association areas in the temporal and frontal lobes.

There is now much evidence that the HF plays a key role in certain kinds of learning and memory. Lesions restricted to the hippocampus proper produce amnesia i.e. impaired memory without perceptible reductions in intelligence that is "shallower" than one that results from damage to the entire HF. The HF appears to mediate short-term memory as isolated damage to it does not seem to erase older ones from a few days ago although it prevents the learning of new material.

Memories can be roughly distinguished into two kinds: declarative or explicit, which relates to the memory of events and facts, while the other called non-declarative or implicit, has to do with the development of skills and habits. It has been found that only the declarative type depends critically on the integrity of the medial temporal lobe. For non-declarative memory, the basal ganglia, cerebellum and regions of the neocortex seem to be more important.

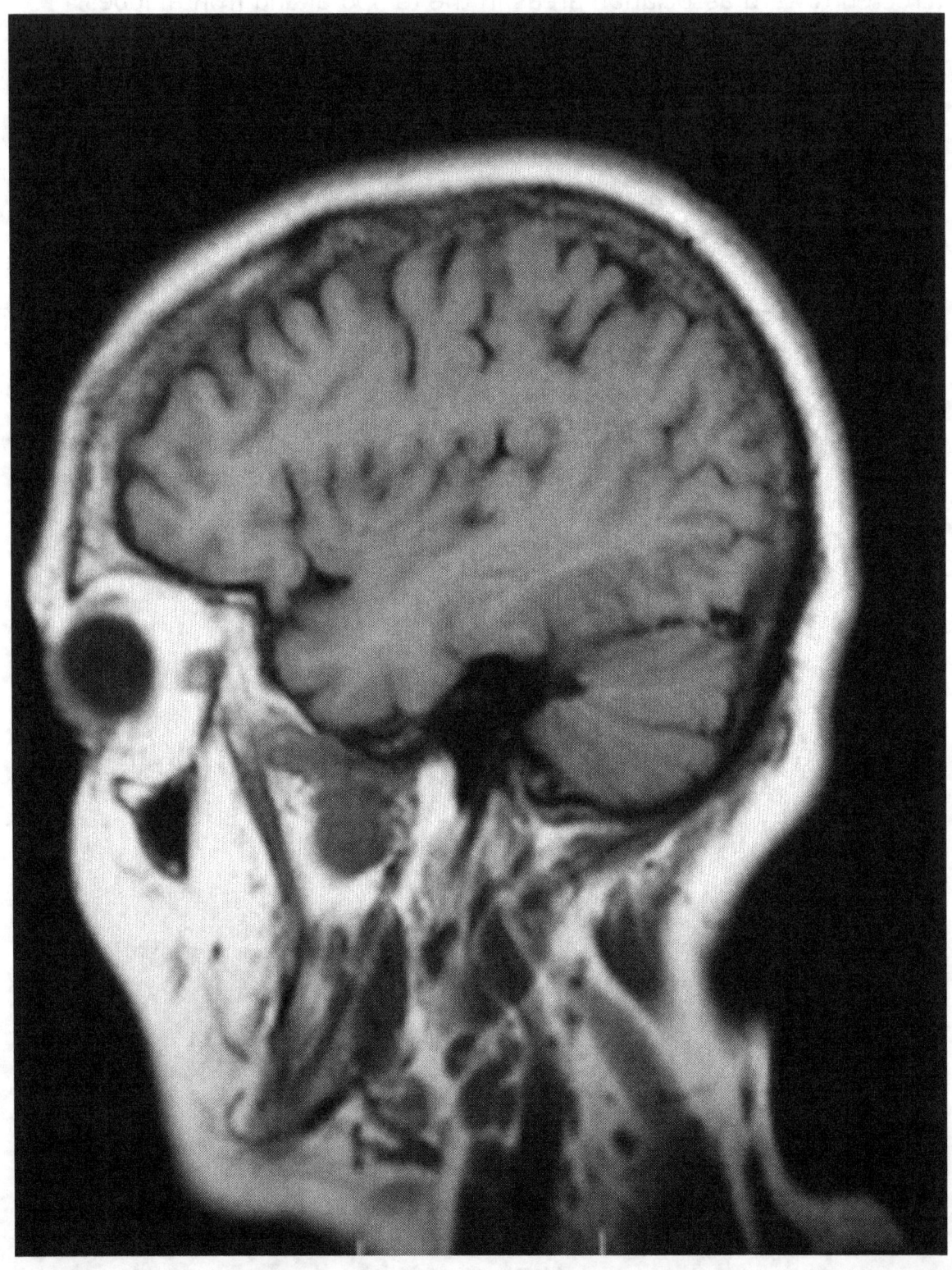

MRI image of sagittal section through Head & Neck

The Prefrontal Cortex (PFC)

In humans, the prefrontal cortex constitutes a massive network that links the brain's motor, perceptual and limbic regions. It occupies nearly half of the entire frontal lobe. There are extensive projections to the PFC from almost all regions of the parietal and temporal cortices and even some from the prestriate regions of the occipital cortex. Subcortical structures including the basal ganglia, cerebellum and various brainstem nuclei project indirectly to the PFC via the thalamus.

Indeed, almost all cortical and subcortical areas influence the PFC either directly or within a few synapses. The PFC also sends reciprocal connections to most areas that project to it including the premotor and motor ones. The PFC has many projections to the contralateral hemisphere; not only to the homologous prefrontal areas via the corpus callosum but also bilateral projections to the premotor and subcortical region. From these neuroanatomical considerations, we can safely assume that the PFC is in an excellent position to coordinate cognitive processing across wide regions of the CNS.

Goal-Oriented Behavior

Our actions are not aimless nor are they entirely dictated by events and stimuli immediately at hand. We choose to act because we want to accomplish goals, to gratify personal needs. These goals dwell within a hierarchy and the ability to form a coherent plan of action is taken as a sign of intelligence and sentience.

In the last fifteen years or so, we have witnessed a burgeoning interest in possible executive functions of the anterior cingulate (AC) cortex. Buried deep in the frontal lobes and characterized by a primitive cytoarchitecture, this neural structure was long assumed to be a component of the Limbic system mediating autonomic responses to pain or threatening situations.

Whereas functional roles for most cortical regions were assigned based on behavioral problems associated with neurological deficits, interest in the AC has been inspired by serendipitous activations found in this region during PET studies. These findings have led to a re-conceptualization of this area as part of the attentional hierarchy. In this view, the AC occupies an upper rung on the hierarchy, playing a key role in coordinating activity across attentional systems.

Complex actions or what is known nowadays as multi-tasking requires that we shift from one sub-goal to another in a coordinated manner. Task-switching experiments have been devised to examine this aspect of executive control. The SAS (supervisory attentional system) or the great Seer, a psychological model of executive control has been invoked to specify some of the key situations in which control operations would be useful.

Although the SAS is usually sketched out in this model as a single entity, it is unlikely that a single neural structure would mediate the complex multi-tasking taking place in real-life scenarios. It would be more plausible to expect that the functions embodied in the SAS are part of a distributed network i.e. a set of neural regions that interact or "share" information facilitating goal-oriented behavior. Evidence suggests that the PFC plays a central role in this function.

Another thing, something in the brain has to monitor "progress" within this multi-tasking behavior, so that a "flow" or sequence can be achieved. This so-called cognitive monitor or *directorial homunculus* seems to lie within the AC. It shows activity on a PET scan only when a novel task is being performed but remains quiet during mundane or routine events. However, the poor temporal resolution of these scans makes it difficult to distinguish between functions associated with activations in the cingulate, lateral prefrontal cortex or disparate posterior foci in the two hemispheres.

Some researchers have sought to identify the source and time course of these temporal events by using event-related potential (ERP) waveforms obtained during simulated multi-task tests in the lab. The PET foci constrained how the generators were modeled.

The first difference was observed about 180 msec after the onset of the task and was attributed to a single generator in the AC. About 30 msec later, a second generator was localized in the lateral PFC in the left hemisphere. Finally, around 620 msec after stimulus onset, a third generator was linked to the posterior cortex of the left hemisphere. The time course fits well with the general picture gleaned from other studies.

We can hypothesize that the initial cingulate activity reflects the allocation of attentional resources to these novel stimuli. The cingulate may establish a *node* in the working memory system of the lateral PFC to hold representations retrieved from the longer-term memory stores held within the posterior cortex. As processing spreads, we can see how a monitoring system can help ensure the successful interaction between working and long-term memory in goal-oriented behavior.

Cognition is "synthesized" from activity at many essential nodes spread around the two cerebral hemispheres and cannot be attributed to one single region or neural network.

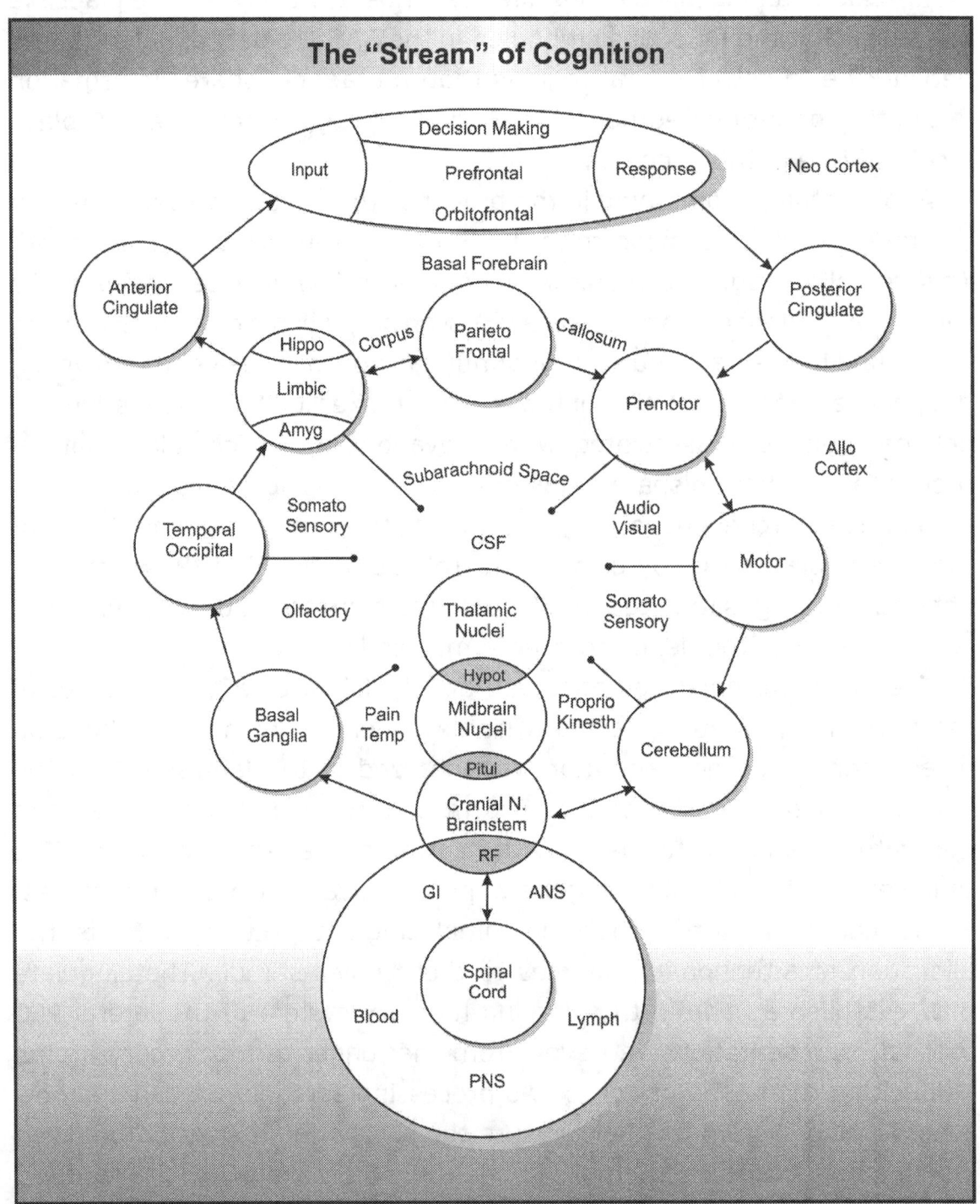

Ilustration of the "Stream" of Cognition

Hemispheric Lateralization & Human Uniqueness

From the perspective of natural selection, by which organisms acquire specific adaptations, one would assume that the two cerebral hemispheres would not function identically. After all, one does not need two speech centers or two places to store a memory of the same face. Once a region of the brain has evolved a functional specialization, there would seem to be no need to duplicate it in another region.

However, the cerebral organization suggests that duplication rather than unilateral specialization is the rule. The two hemispheres are much more similar to each other in function than one may think. The differences only surface at a more subtle level of analysis. Each hemisphere's visual areas are devoted to representing the shapes and colors of objects and their primary specialization relates to the object's position: Is the object on the left side of space or the right?

What is more, the motor cortices are roughly mirror images of each other, both in structure and function. While each cortex can be represented by a motor homunculus of the body, it is dominated by fibers that project to muscles on the opposite side of the body. Evolution could have utilized the available cerebral space in a completely different way.

Visual functions could have been isolated in the left hemisphere and motor projections to both limbs could have originated in the right. Yet, selective pressures appear to have favored a cerebral organization that reflects structural properties of the world and the organism. The world's spatial structure is reflected in our biology.

The hemispheric specializations are best conceived as superimposed on this fundamental symmetry. In some instances, specializations may have evolved because there was an advantage in having a single system devoted to a certain process. For example, one hypothesis postulates that speech production became strongly lateralized because of the need to communicate at rapid rates. Transcortical processing and integration take time and may slow down complicated articulatory gestures. Indeed, lateralization may underlie stuttering because of the two parallel systems that compete for control of speech output.

Others argue that hemispheric specializations evolved because of the inherent advantages in having nonidentical forms of representation. Homologous visual areas perform related operations but differently enough that the resultant nonidentical representations are imbued with unique advantages in performing certain tasks.

This does not mean that these tasks are strictly localized, that language functions are restricted to the left or spatial ones to the right. Not only does the normal performance of these tasks require distributed operations that may span both hemispheres but also usually, both hemispheres contain the essential machinery for performing the task.

This organization help explain why patients with large unilateral lesions that damage 25% of the cortical tissue on one side still display an amazing capacity for recovery. Evidence that is even more dramatic comes from patients with isolated cerebral hemispheres, a condition that arises after a so-called split-brain operation. Because this radical operation remarkably preserves function, such patients are invaluable for giving us clues to subtle functional asymmetries and basic capabilities of each cerebral hemisphere.

Research on brain laterality has provided extensive insights into the organization of the human cortex. The surgical disconnection of the cerebral hemispheres (split brain) has produced an extraordinary opportunity to study which cognitive and perceptual processes, are cortical in nature and which, subcortical. Researchers have discovered that visual perceptual and tactile-patterned information; for instance, remain strictly lateralized to one hemisphere following sectioning of the corpus callosum.

When the corpus callosum is fully sectioned, little or no perceptual interaction takes place between the now isolated hemispheres. Surgical cases where callosal section is limited or part of the callosum is spared have enabled investigators to examine specific functions mediated by regions.

For instance, when the splenium, the posterior area of the callosum that links the occipital lobe is spared, visual information is transferred normally.

The patterns, colors and linguistic info presented anywhere in either field can be matched with the info presented to the other half of the brain. However, the patients show no evidence of inter-hemispheric transfer of tactile info from objects felt by them. These observations are consistent with other human and animal data showing that major callosum subdivisions are organized into functional zones: posterior ones mediate visual info and the anterior ones transfer auditory and tactile info.

The anterior region of the callosum is involved in higher-order transfer of semantic info i.e. the patient is able to name stimuli presented in the left VF following a resection limited to the posterior callosal region. Upon sectioning of the anterior callosum, this capacity ceased.

By testing each disconnected hemisphere, one can assess the different capacities each might possess. While some claims are exaggerated, there are marked differences between the two halves. The most prominent lateralized function in the human brain is the left hemisphere's capacity for language and speech.

The second primary task domain studied in split-brain subjects is visuo-spatial processing. Here the simple task of arranging some red and white blocks to match those of a given pattern demonstrates poor performance by the left hemisphere while the right one excels.

However, if a picture of the block design pattern is lateralized, each hemisphere can easily find the match from a series of pictures. Moreover, since each hand is sufficiently dexterous, the crucial link must be in the mapping of the sensory message onto the capable motor system.

After the human cerebral hemispheres are disconnected, the verbal IQ of the patient remains intact and although there may be some deficits in free recall capacity, the problem-solving ability of the left hemisphere appears unaffected. However, the right hemisphere seems incapable of higher-order thought processes providing compelling evidence that cortical cell number by itself cannot fully explain human intelligence.

Attentional mechanisms, however, can involve other subcortical systems. Taken together, cortical disconnection produces two independent sensory information-processing systems that call upon a common attentional resource system in carrying out perceptual tasks.

Split-brain studies also reveal a complex mosaic of mental processes that enter into human cognition. As noted above, the two hemispheres do not represent information in an identical manner as evidenced by the fact that each one has developed its own *repertoire* of specialized capacities.

In the vast majority of individuals, the left hemisphere is clearly dominant for language and speech and seems to possess a uniquely human capacity to interpret behavior or to construct "theories" about the relationship between perceived events and feelings. Right-hemisphere superiority, on the other hand, can be seen in tasks such as facial recognition and attentional monitoring. Both hemispheres are likely to be involved in the performance of any complex task, but with each contributing in a special manner.

All models of normal language comprehension have to begin with the problem of how words are represented. Understanding spoken language and understanding written language share some processes but there are also some striking differences in how spoken and written inputs are analyzed by the brain.

The input signal in spoken language is very different from that in written ones. Whereas for a reader it is immediately clear that the letters on a page are the physical signals of importance, a listener is confronted by a series of sounds intermingled with others in the environment. He has to identify and distinguish the relevant speech signals from other "noise".

Numerous studies suggest that the superior temporal (ST) cortex is important in mediating sound perception in humans whereas some PET and fMRI studies that have looked at reading of words and pseudowords (sound like words but have no inherent meaning) found middle temporal gyrus activations. This may imply that reading can and often does activate phonological information.

For written input, readers must recognize a visual pattern, which may vary across different writing systems. The symbols used are abstract representations that do not resemble what they represent. The actual identification of such orthographic units may take place in the occipital-temporal regions of the left hemisphere.

The inherent complexity of the language system does hamper the elucidation of its structure and neural mechanisms and so the struggle to clarify them remains one of the great scientific challenges currently facing cognitive neuroscience.

Nonhuman primates also have differences in hemispheric structure or function. In anatomical studies of Old World monkeys and apes, we find asymmetries similar to those of humans. For example, the sylvian fissure shows a greater upward slope in the right hemisphere and there is a similar forward skewedness of the right hemisphere. Whether these anatomical asymmetries are associated with behavioral specializations remains obscure and the case for hemispheric specialization in nonhuman primates is not compelling.

Much unlike humans, the nonhuman primates do not show a predominance of right-handedness. Individual animals may display a preference for one hand or the other but there is no consistent trend for the right hand to be favored over the left either when making manual gestures or when fabricating tools.

Perceptual studies provide more provocative indications of parallel asymmetrical functions in humans and other primates. The rhesus monkeys are superior in making tactile discriminations of shape when using the left hand as in humans. What is more impressive is that split-brain monkeys show hemispheric interactions comparable to those observed in humans on visual perception tasks. In a face recognition test, the monkeys have a right hemisphere advantage whereas in a line orientation task, the monkeys have a left hemisphere edge.

Complementary studies on patients with focal brain lesions and normal controls tested with lateralized stimuli and even comparative approaches have underlined not only the presence but also the importance of lateralized processes active in cognition and perception.

Recent work, such as the spatial frequency hypothesis has moved brain laterality research toward a more computational account of hemispherical specialization seeking to explicate the mechanisms underlying many lateralized perceptual phenomena. These theoretical advances are taking the field away from the popular interpretations of cognitive style and providing a scientific basis for these robust processes.

Section 4

Cognition vs. Consciousness

The Birth of Sentience

Each species has evolved its own *modus operandi* based on the complexity of their nervous system. This simple fact implies that even though all the various species inhabit the same world, they tend to interact with that environment differently. Bees 'see' in UV light, snakes sense infra red radiation, birds navigate using cues from the Earth's magnetic field, fish possess sense organs sensitive to vibrations in the water while dogs have hyperacute smelling and hearing abilities.

So when in evolution did *consciousness* first appear?

Well, it all depends on how you define consciousness!

Simple *awareness* of the surroundings and environment arose quite early in animal evolution. Internal homeostatic mechanisms dependent on numerous sense organs were in place by the bacterial or amoeba stage of evolution.

This was followed by 'avoidance and predatory mechanisms' where the organism either fled the scene or attacked, depending on how its sensory organs 'assessed' the situation. There was no true 'understanding' or 'insight' here. In Humphrey's words, they "went about their lives, deeply ignorant of an inner explanation of their own behaviour."

Next came 'intelligence', where the animal is now capable of not only *assessing*, but is also able to mount a *graded* response via a true analysis of the situation. Analogous to the action of a dimmer switch, intelligence comes gradually in increments and degrees, with increasing complexity of the underlying neural assembly.

In the so-called higher mammals and primates, innate intelligence evolved into a *true* understanding of consequences and a *rudimentary* concept of self. As any pet owner will attest, kittens will rush up to a mirror as if looking for its playmate. Many birds continue to carry-on and peck at their image as if confronted by a hostile rival. Even monkeys clearly fail to 'understand' that the reflection is their own.

The great apes, on the other hand, gorillas, chimps, orangs and humans, quickly realize this and recognizing themselves in the mirror, begin to 'inspect' various hidden attributes of their body. Interestingly enough, human babies, *below* two years of age also fail to recognize themselves in a mirror. Teenagers, on the other hand, cannot get enough of their reflection and are always seeking out mirrored surfaces in shopping malls.

According to Dennett, a cognitive scientist at Tufts University, sometime during the second year or so, babies begin to follow another person's direction of gaze rather than their pointing finger. Numerous experiments demonstrate that between the ages of three and five, humans develop a so-called 'theory of mind' i.e. begin to understand other people's behavior as 'intentional'.

They attribute mental states to others or to themselves that govern hope, fears, wants and needs. This aspect of consciousness is absent in most other advanced mammals and is seen as a very powerful 'tool' for understanding, manipulating and predicting the world around us. It also heralds the birth of true self-consciousness.

It is plausible that some animals notably mammals possess some but not necessarily all features of the consciousness spectrum via their sensorium tailor-made to navigate efficiently in their ecological niche. Many people that have pets and work closely with animals intuitively assume that they have their own flavor of subjective states. To believe otherwise is not only presumptuous, but flies in the face of experimental evidence for the continuity of behavioral patterns between animals and humans.

This is particularly true for monkeys and apes, whose behavior, development and brain structure are remarkably similar to those of humans. In fact, one of the best ways to study stimulus awareness today relies on correlating neuronal responses of trained monkeys to their behavior.

Obviously, humans do differ fundamentally from all organisms in their ability to speak. True language enables *Homo sapiens* to represent and disseminate arbitrarily complex concepts. Unfortunately, the primacy of language in the human social milieu has given rise to a belief among philosophers, linguists and other theoreticians that consciousness is impossible without a true language and that therefore, only humans can feel and introspect.

While this may be partially true, most evidence from split-brain patients, autistic children, evolutionary studies and diverse animal behavior observations does suggest that most of the "higher" mammals do cognate and experience various degrees of pain and emotions. At present, it is unknown to what extent conscious perception is common to all animals. It is possible that consciousness correlates to some extent with the complexity of its nervous system.

Squids, bees, fruit flies and even roundworms are all capable of fairly sophisticated behaviors. Perhaps they too possess some level of awareness, feel pain, experience pleasure and plan foraging routines. It would be contrary to evolutionary continuity to believe that consciousness is unique to humans. As we will see throughout this book, the human mind does share some basic properties with animal minds.

Stereotaxic studies, done on animal subjects with microelectrodes reveal segregated cortical neighborhoods whose neurons are specialized to carry out different jobs. For instance, neurons in one occipital-temporal region are particularly sensitive to the color or hue of stimuli. Neurons in the MT region detect movement in the environment whereas neurons of the posterior parietal cortex program fine eye movements to track them. Clinical observations of patients suffering from mild neurological deficits reinforce the view that particular regions of the cerebral cortex subserve specific functions.

Cortical areas in the back of the brain are organized in a loosely hierarchical manner with at least a dozen levels, each one subordinate to the one above it. When a group of neurons within one of these regions receives a strong driving input from lower in the hierarchy, the neurons send their output to another area or group located higher in the hierarchy. Feedback loops abound and numerous 'short-cuts' are present within this structured assembly producing a flexible "coalition", if you will, rather than a rigid hierarchy.

The incoming sensory information is also not usually enough to lead to an unambiguous interpretation. In such cases, then, the cortical networks fill in. They make their best guess, given the incomplete information. This filling-in occurs throughout the brain and guides much of animal or for that matter, human behavior. Any visual scene gives rise to widespread activity across the brain.

Coalitions of neurons, coding for different objects in the world out there, compete with each other i.e. one coalition strives to suppress or inhibit others, vying for a subjective response. This is particularly true in the higher centers of the cortex. Paying attention to an event or object biases this competition in its favor leading to the emergence of a winner. The activity associated with the winning coalition corresponds to the conscious state.

Usually only a single coalition survives but in many cases when the neuronal representations do not overlap, several may coexist alongside for a while. The losing coalitions do not, however, lie down and die. Like inveterate politicians, they continue to remain active and influence the cortical hierarchy, jockeying to win the next election.

The essential *difference* between the twin processes of cognition and consciousness, as I see it, using the terminology of today, is the difference between a *tangible* computer system and *virtual* cyberspace. The brain along with its neuronal elements symbolizes a modern computer and the intricate "web" constructed by it to do it's computation in, is what we call consciousness.

Just as the computer requires *cyberspace* to function within, the brain constructs this elaborate virtual workspace, to perform its duty.

Does that mean that consciousness is a mere *epiphenomenon* brought about by a functioning brain or complex neural network?

I'm not sure.

Is it some kind of *metaphoric* space, stage or Cartesian Theater within which cognition occurs?

Possibly.

So where is this place or space in the real Einsteinian SpaceTime continuum?

It is hard to explain or pin down, just like cyberspace. Nobody really knows what or where it is but everyone works in it whenever any computer terminal is used. It is definitely not *real* physical 3D space but *virtual* or made-up space, a figment of our imagination!

However, this is where all the "mental stuff" takes place: trances, meditation, OBEs, NDEs, paranormal phenomena, ESP etc., etc.

The Human Mind

There is much disagreement over how and when consciousness first appeared on Earth. Some believe that its appearance was gradual, increasing like a *dimmer switch,* if you will, with each increment in brain size. Others, like the pan-psychists, believe the entire universe is conscious, although there are degrees of it ranging from the simple (rocks, bacteria and viruses) to increasingly complex (animals and primates). In this view, consciousness itself came long before biological evolution began and gradually evolved into the higher forms.

Some believe that life and consciousness are inseparable and emerged together four *billion* years ago. Others think that consciousness requires a complex nervous system and that it must have evolved along with the increasing complexity of brains. Finally, there are those who feel that consciousness dates from the increasingly social *milieu* of our early ancestors, circa two *million* years ago, which induced them to build novel skills of understanding, predicting and manipulating the behaviors of others.

An interesting implication of this hypothesis is that only intelligent and highly social creatures are conscious i.e. most creatures prior to such creatures through much of the Earth's history were *not* conscious at all. Their 'brains' processed information from the sense organs without 'thinking' and their bodies acted to avoid fear and hunger, without their 'minds' being conscious of any accompanying emotions.

How does the brain *convert* sensory signals into a coherent perception of the world out there?

Considering the complexity of the nervous system, it is amazing how easily we take in all the familiar sights and sounds of the neighborhood to form a coherent precept. In the next few pages, we will explore the big picture, if you will, of the cognitive neuroscience of perception.

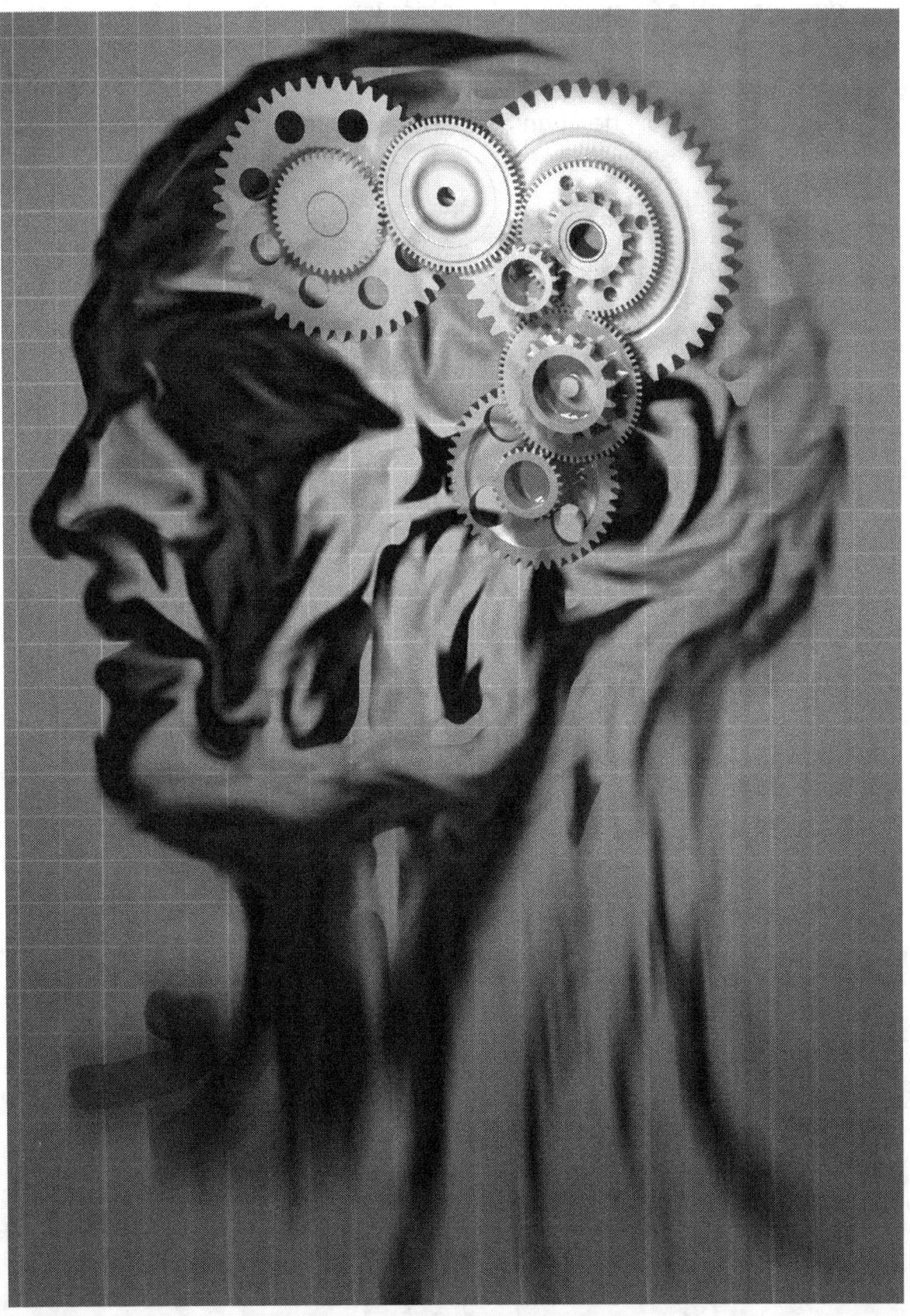

The Human Cognitive Mind

Human Awareness and Sensory Information

A human being's awareness of the world is mediated by numerous physiological mechanisms, involved in the processing and organization of afferent or sensory stimuli impinging upon the central nervous system. Initially, the incoming stimulus energy evokes *action potentials* within individual nerve fibers.

The action potential has characteristics determined only by the properties of the neuron, independent of the characteristics of the exciting stimulus. It is in a coded form. The code represents information from the external world, differing vastly from the actual incoming stimulus it seems to be representing. For example, the eye does not really form an inverted image of the outside world on the retina as most people believe.

Instead, myriad receptors in the ten layers of the retina break down the visual cues into a steady stream of coded electrical impulses. These flow through the million odd neurons of each optic nerve to the thalamus (LGN) for further processing. This *edited* information then passes on to the primary visual cortex layers where it is organized into bits and pieces of a complex puzzle.

A database of memories and prior experiences are meticulously accessed via a massive network of reciprocating 'association' fibers that infuse the 'picture' with emotions and feelings. All this information now flows into the 'executive' branch of the brain, which helps us 'register' the scene playing out in the outside world and grant it 'recognition'. Only 500 milliseconds have transpired between first setting eyes on an object and recognition!

Afferent information may or may not have a conscious correlate i.e. it may or may not give rise to a conscious awareness of the physical world.

Afferent information that does not have a conscious correlate is called sensory information and the conscious experience of objects and events of the external world, which we acquire from the neural processing of sensory information, is called perception.

Intuitively it may seem that the sensory systems of our body operate like some our more familiar electrical equipment used in interpersonal communications, for example, a telephone. However, there are some essential differences. A phone changes sound waves into electrical impulses and back into sound waves.

Our hearing system changes the sound waves into *graded* action potentials, which are processed by the brain as *sound*. The brain does not physically translate the code into sound waves. Currently, just as in the visual system example above, we have no clear understanding of how these coded action potentials are perceived as conscious sensations.

Information about the external world and internal body environment exists in different energy forms e.g. pressure, temperature, light, sound, smell etc., but only specific receptors can deal with them. Even though any one receptor is usually more responsive to one specific stimulus modality, several different energy forms can activate virtually all of them, if the stimulus intensity is sufficient, or if the receptor is unusually sensitive.

The rest of the nervous system can extract meaning only from the graded or action potential in which it is encoded. Several different kinds of information (stimulus modality, intensity and localization) are conveyed in code to the CNS.

All incoming afferent information is subject to extensive control before it reaches the higher levels of the CNS and much of it may be reduced or even abolished by inhibitory input from other neurons. Our actual perception of the events around us often involves areas of the brain other than the primary sensory cortex. Systems for controlling attention include the parietal lobe, temporal cortex, frontal cortex and various subcortical structures.

Information from the primary areas achieves further elaboration through the neural activity of nerve fibers relaying information from cortical association areas. These perform higher mental functions like providing contextual information memory, recall of past circumstantial information and collating it into a more 'personalized' version of the event. All of us put great trust in our sensory-perceptual processes despite the inevitable modification and editing we know that tends to exist in the CNS.

Some of the factors known to distort our perceptions of the real world can be:

Receptor-adaptation to certain recurrent stimuli, either due to receptor fatigue or personal disregard.

Or, confounding factors such as emotions, personality and social background, influencing perception,

Or, not all information entering the CNS is giving rise to conscious sensations.

Or, incompleteness of the real picture due to the lack of suitable receptors for many regions of the electromagnetic spectrum.

Thus, it appears obvious that the twin processes of transmitting data through the nervous system and interpreting it, cannot be separated. The information is processed at each synaptic level of the afferent pathways and there is no one point along its sojourn when it can be interpreted as becoming suddenly 'conscious'.

Perception has many levels and it seems that the many separate stages follow a sort of neurological *hierarchy*, with the more complex ones receiving input only after it has undergone processing by the more elementary systems. Every synapse along the lengthy pathway adds an element of organization and seems to contribute to the overall sensory experience.

Some people feel that we are 'not ready' to undertake a systematic approach to the study of Consciousness as we need to know more about brain functions in non-conscious phenomena first.

I agree.

Others feel that the problem of consciousness is not really a *scientific* problem at all but safely left to philosophers and theologians. Still others remain skeptical that we cannot give a biological account of consciousness as no scientist or science could ever explain our first-person subjective responses to things 'out there' in the real world.

Though the current assault on the field of studies on consciousness and *Mind* phenomena is promising, the scientists are barely scratching at the surface of the complex neurological processes that underlie human awareness.

Many 'prominent' neuroscientists equipped with the latest gadgets of modern medical technology and the highest academic 'diplomas' have devoted endless hours, probing into the deepest recesses of the neocortex with the sole purpose of fleshing out the physiological mechanisms, they feel may 'nail down' the basic precepts of consciousness in humans.

Some camps feel that if they could figure out how the brain processes visual input from a colored object to construct the actual visual experience of color then they could easily extrapolate this finding to explain sounds, tastes, smells and finally consciousness.

Others prefer a more *holistic* approach. They want to find out how the brain produces this *field* of qualitative, unified subjectivity that we know as consciousness.

What is the essential difference between the conscious and unconscious brain?

As we have seen earlier in the book, the neo-cortical gray matter of the human brain is a highly integrated system consisting of a six-to-nine layered 'sheet' of about 10 billion neurons with upto a trillion synapses. Intuitively, all the neuroscientists have converged on the brain as the only anatomical entity that could possibly mediate and sustain consciousness.

In their view, the term consciousness includes two distinct concepts:

(1)   States of Consciousness (SOC), and

(2)   Conscious experience i.e. thoughts and emotions, during the SOC.

In my opinion, they are looking for it in all the 'wrong' places. The human CNS, like the Empire State building, is the culmination of a long lineage of biological architecture and mental refinement. We need to keep in mind that the CNS *evolved*. It was not created *en masse* by some supernatural Agency or Creative Force. In order to gain a basic understanding of 'dwellings' one needs to study an animal 'shelter' first.

We need to go 'down' the phylo-genetic scale of earthly organisms and 'decide' when *true* consciousness made its debut; whether it is at the cellular cytoskeleton level in Amoebas, or further up when the *notochord* (primitive central neural axis) first appeared, in Chordates.

In a unicellular organism, like the bacterium or even the amoeba, all these neurological states are induced within the confines of its cell wall (triggered by various chemical 'messengers'), analogous to the same 'one room shelter' serving as a kitchen, living room or bedroom depending on the situational demand.

Cells are in a way more complex than an embryo. The reason is that the network of interactions between proteins and DNA within any individual cell has many more components and is consequently much more complicated than the interactions between individual cells of a developing embryo. For example, when a cell receives a signal at its membrane from another cell, it precipitates an entire cascade of protein-protein interaction, which may lead to the opening of an ion channel or a certain cluster of genes being switched on/off or the abrupt extension of a pseudopod that propels the amoeba out of danger.

Any given cell at a given time is expressing hundreds if not thousands of different genes much of which may reflect an intrinsic program of activity, independent of external signals. It is this degree of complexity, which determines how cells respond to various stimuli. This state can reflect the cell's development history – cells have good memories – and so different cells can respond to the same signal in very different ways. Numerous researchers have noticed many examples of the same signals being used repeatedly by different cells at different stages of embryonic development with different biological outcomes.

The evolution of multicellular forms of life is the result of changes in development, which in turn is due to changes in genes that control cell behavior in the embryo. Nothing in Biology makes sense unless viewed in the light of evolution. Certainly, it would be quite a challenge to make sense of many aspects of development without an evolutionary perspective.

For example, despite different modes of very early development, all vertebrate embryos develop through a rather similar *phylotypic* stage after which their development diverges again. This shared stage, which occurs after neurulation and the formation of the somites, is a *fundamental* characteristic in the development of all vertebrates.

The neural tube generates a large number of different neuronal and glial cell types. In both the brain and spinal cord, all neurons and glia arise from a proliferative layer of epithelial cells lining the lumen of the neural tube. Once formed, a neuron never divides and migrates to its designated area. Growth cones at the tip of the extending axon guide it to its destination. Filopodial activity at the growth cone is influenced by environmental factors such as contact with the substratum, other cells or subtle gradients in cell-surface molecules (chemotaxis).

The mammalian cerebral cortex is organized into six layers (I – VI), numbered from the surface in. Each layer contains cells of distinctive shapes and connections. The identity of a cortical neuron is specified *before* it begins its migration. The layer to which neurons migrate after their birth in the proliferative layer is related to the time of its birth. Thus, there is an inside-outside sequence of neural differentiation in the neural tube, which gives rise to the cerebral cortex and other layered brain structures like the cerebellum.

The vertebrate visual system has been the subject of intense scrutiny for many years and the highly organized almost *hierarchical* projection of neurons from the eye to the brain is one of the best models we have to show how specific neural connections are made. A characteristic feature of the vertebrate brain is the presence of *topographic maps* i.e. the neurons from one region project in an ordered manner to one region of the brain, so that nearest-neighbor relations are maintained.

The brain scientists were initially quite intrigued by this anatomical hierarchy but then realized that analogous to the layered structures found in a large corporation, such an architecture permits the 'higher' cortical regions to easily detect 'discrepancies' in the 'lower' ones.

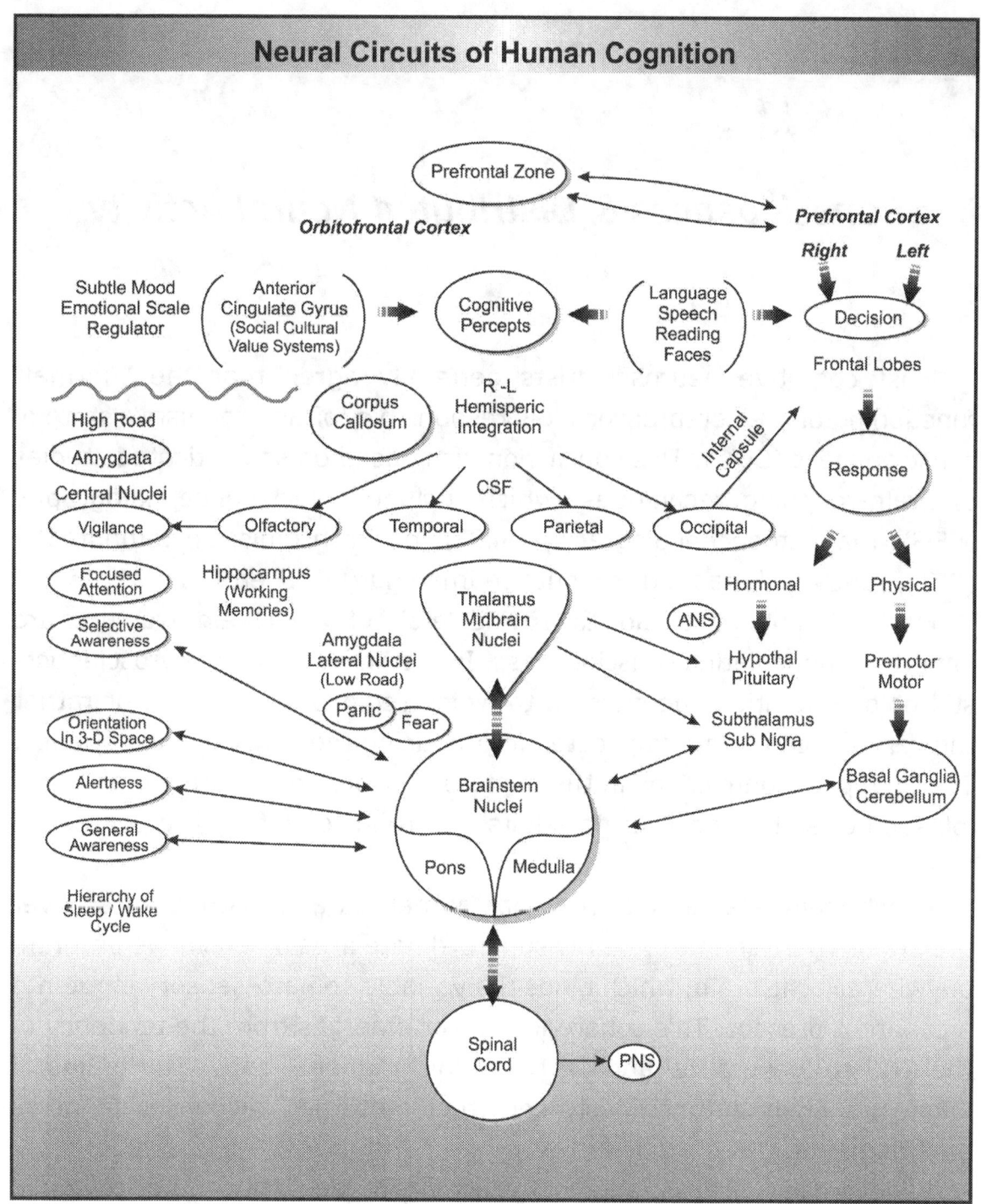

Neural Circuits of Human Cognition

Consciousness & Distributed Neural Activity

Most cognitive neuroscientists generally agree that the "normal" functioning of the cerebral cortex is responsible for an organism's state of consciousness (SOC). This conclusion was based on sophisticated studies of brain-mapping techniques, which included electroencephalography (EEG), magnetoencephalography (MEG), positron emission tomography (PET), functional magnetic resonance imaging (fMRI) etc.

Many attempts were made to provide details of which brain structures are important in mediating consciousness. In fact, modern-day neuroscientists still hold contentious debates as to which regions of the brain or rather the cerebral cortex are implicated in producing the conscious experience. The 'mapped' connections in the somato-sensory cortex are variable and 'plastic i.e. soft-wired even in adults and tend to shift in the context of use.

Functionally specialized areas are numerous and distributed all over the brain. There seems to be NO superordinate area or executive program anywhere in the brain, which binds the variable somato-sensory input into a coherent precept. This coherent precept emerges from the tendency of the CNS to 'generalize' and to 'fill-in' informational gaps. The brains of 'higher' animals autonomously construct patterned responses to novel environments.

Widespread synchronization of the activity of widely distributed neuronal groups occurs via a vast network of reciprocal inter-connections following the law of 'weighted averages'. The collated information flows across the somato-sensory cortex via the ANS (autonomic nervous system), the RF, the Limbic circuit, Basal Ganglia and the Thalamus.

188

The graded amplification of 'recruited' neural groups results in an evoked potential after a 500 *millisecond* pause, which represents the time interval required for the collated information to 'transform' into a cognitive precept. The reader needs to keep in mind that there is NO fixed instructional plan or *homunculus* lingering in the brain or CNS.

The ability to create a 'scene' by correlating the somato-sensory input to its internal memory maps gives rise to the emergence of *primary* consciousness. These maps are built up from integrated signals arising from the entire CNS/ANS systems, which provide a central referential basis for primary consciousness.

Consciousness is an active, multi-tiered process and tends to be *hierarchical* in nature. All the higher-order levels of consciousness rest on the primary one and confer the ability to think, imagine the future, recall the past and *be* conscious of *being* conscious. It is normally unitary but capable of shifting through a multitude of inner states instantly and by choice.

A functional cluster of neurons embedded all along the cerebro-spinal axis brings about the current state of consciousness. The changes of neural activity along this axis give rise to the entire range of subjective precepts via the individual's experiential repertoire and non-representational memory stores. The Edelman-Tononi team, after reviewing the vast field of neurological and neurophysiological evidence promulgated certain conclusions.

First, conscious processes are typically associated with distributed changes in activity in the thalamocortical system.

Second, distributed changes in neural activity associated with conscious experience require integration through 'reentrant' interactions that are both rapid and effective.

Finally, these interactions are associated with conscious reports if they are highly differentiated but not if they are uniform or homogenous.

These observations suggest that the neurological processes mediating consciousness are highly integrated but continually changing i.e. in a dynamic flux. Variable inputs from the sensorimotor systems monitoring the environment constantly update the SOC in *real* time.

Hobson's Brain-Mind Paradigm

Basic principles

An American psychiatrist and sleep researcher Allan Hobson developed the AIM model, which depicts the three states of consciousness in 3D space, by using data from behavioral and physiological studies. It allows for any state of the brain-mind to be positioned within it. Adding Time as a fourth dimension permits cycling through the various sleep-wake states and provides a visual representation scheme for placing them in the context of the numerous neurotransmitter systems implicated in mediating the SOC's.

The Brain-Mind (B-M) is a unified system i.e. No Brain, No Mind.

Normal consciousness is a B-M state in which the Brain is aware of its own physical state.

There are normally three B-M states: Alert, Awake and Asleep, controlled by the Reticular Activating System (RAS) of the Spinal cord and Brainstem.

The RAS controls and modulates these B-M states via a complex neuro-chemical system during an approximate 24-hr circadian biorhythm mediated by the Pineal gland. This system comprises of the amino-cholinergic axis located in the central aspect of the brainstem and the circulating cerebro-spinal fluid (CSF).

There is NO *single* area in the brain responsible for consciousness.

Consciousness, by definition, is not a tangible entity or an epiphenomenon 'produced' by the 'working' brain. It represents an *active* process that requires the participation of many cortical components scattered throughout the brainstem and cortex.

It is a *biological* feature of the Central Nervous System (CNS). A great deal of our thinking proceeds without conscious awareness. Consciousness is an *emergent* property of the CNS after it has reached a *critical* level of complexity. Synchronous 'waves' of 40 Hz every 12.5 seconds recorded on an EEG link and integrate various cortical areas into one functioning whole. The Thalamus seems to be a key area in generating this synchrony.

The brain-mind seems to traverse through the nREM and REM states in part to reinforce and reorganize memory. Reinforcement occurs via consolidation e.g. an experience that we had during the day reactivates as we dream. This advances them from short-term into long-term memory, perhaps mediated by Ach, which is omnipresent during sleep.

REM sleep is a time when the brain-mind does not have to accept new data but at the same time has unlimited access to all the existing action files of our motor program. In short, our memory is consolidated within a framework of motor programs within the brain.

When we decide to go somewhere, we voluntarily initiate movement sequences. Once they begin, though, they are so automatic that they no longer require our conscious supervision. Walking, running, sprinting are gaits controlled by the brainstem motor-pattern generators.

All we have to do is flip a command switch in our cortex and our brainstem coordinates the motion. This is a top-down process: our brain thinks about walking and the centers for gait control situated in the brainstem and spinal cord spring into action.

In cases of emergency, we react automatically first and then a split second later realize the danger and feel afraid. In these cases, the brainstem signals to react precede our conscious thoughts. These acts are bottom-up processes.

Whether or not the motor-pattern generators are under voluntary (top-down) or automatic (bottom-up) control depends on our state of consciousness (SOC). The gait control circuits are in the brainstem, intertwined with the same networks that govern brain-mind states. These circuits are hard-wired into the brain by periodic activation, which begins *in utero* and click on every time we sleep.

Once we have set the brain-mind in motion, all we have to do is shape and modify this program through accumulated experience. This is what it means to learn. We actively inscribe what we have learned into the dynamic structure of an automatic process.

At some point early in life, the system acquires a rich enough stock of images and thoughts to have conscious awareness. Add a few more and it has enough to be aware of being aware. Once we have this quality of self-awareness, we become human or fully conscious.

Now, in order for us to survive in the world as babies, we need to be born knowing how to do certain things, behaviors that are sort of pre-programmed by the self-activated brain, in REM, long before they are put to the service of survival. This programmed automaticity of brain-mind states also necessarily extends into various other aspects of our mental life. Collectively known as *procedural* knowledge, it emerges spontaneously and naturally when called upon to do so. Every sensory experience, be it veridical or illusory, seems to involve action and belief, movement and concept. Our brain is trained through motion.

Nevertheless, how can we ensure that this experience is built into our system?

Moreover, how can we be sure that this procedure, once built-in stays there for life?

One way would be to have a state (waking) in which we are exposed to new info and another (REM sleep) in which this new data is *integrated* into the whole set of existing programs in the system.

In order for this to happen, the system needs to run automatically for a considerable length of time each day (say 90 minutes of REM sleep). It needs to be fast (six procedures a second, the usual rate of PGO wave signals), run with the clutch disengaged (so that the system does not have to output); and occur in an altered chemical climate (Ach versus Amines).

Of course, a system of such complexity does tend to break down under certain situations, especially if we do not get enough sleep or there are small shifts of balance in the aminergic-cholinergic control system. These deficits or imbalances occur in altered SOCs, fugue states, drug-induced trances and dubious meditations.

Now, if our mind represents all the information in our brain, then this info is either accessible i.e. conscious or inaccessible (non-conscious). It cannot exist in any other mode. In other words, all our thoughts and willed actions are called conscious, whereas the motor programs that control our thinking and movements are termed non-conscious or autonomous.

The information that can move from the nonconscious (nCON) to consciousness (CON) includes much of what we call memory. Memory consists of perceptions that we can call forth as imagery, most of our emotions, instincts and a vast set of procedural talents. What ultimately happens with this information depends on the state of the brain.

To summarize, the intricate workings of the brain-mind and the resulting process of Consciousness are deeply rooted in the laws of Physics and Biochemistry: a rise of the biogenic amines within the body causes the activation of the RAS, which mediates the Wake Cycle. Being awake for the entire day 'weakens' the amines, enabling the cholinergic system to emerge.

The steady increase in cholines causes relaxation of the body, bringing on sleep. The presence of Ach also kicks on the REM sleep, helps initiate dreaming and the final lapse into deep sleep. Once the amines have regrouped, the RAS is gradually *ramped up*, causing us to wake again.

The waking state enables us to etch this information into the permanent memories of our nCON mind. Other so-called altered SOCs of the brain-mind enable this info to travel between the two modes of the B-M system i.e. nCON and CON.

During paradoxical sleep or REM, the firing of cholinergic neurons precipitates the dream state. In other words, a chemical neurotransmitter is able to open up a channel from the non-conscious to the conscious mind. Is there a similar mechanism in place to *descend* from the conscious to the non-conscious?

The Indian yogi seems to think so.

Through a highly focused training of the thought process, the disciplined devotee plugs directly into the neuronal activation patterns of the brain-mind duality. He believes that this enables him to perceive "true" *Reality*. These 'advanced' humans are proof that even though the mind is extremely elusive, embodied in the very depths of the CNS, it is still palpable through the one-pointed focus of introspection reached during the altered SOC of *samadhi*.

Unity of Consciousness

Since so many of neurological studies implicate the immensely diversified brain as being the main organ system mediating our states of consciousness, why do we feel as though there is just one 'mind' experiencing a unified world out there? In other words, there is one constant and undifferentiated self, 'me', perceiving the world through one continuous 'stream' of experiences occurring around 'me'.

Our experiencing self seems to be at the center of everything we are aware of at a given time and to be continuous from one moment to the next. It thus seems to have both unity and continuity: an inner agent that carries out actions, makes decisions, bestows a unique personality to the Self and becomes the sole determinant of your lifestyle.

However, is this perception... false?

Do we really have an underlying, unitary Self, separate from their physical brain (Dualism)?

Or... is it, as the Buddha claimed, that there is no such thing as the Self, but just a name or label given to something that does not exist (Monism)?

Or... we could simply reject the whole idea that consciousness is a unified entity and call it as being just a big delusion, induced by the machinations of *Maya Jahl* (Web of Delusion)?

These opposing views capture a fundamental split in the way most people think about the nature of Self.

Popper and Eccles argue that the *mind* plays an active role in selecting, reading out and integrating neural activity, molding it into a unified whole according to its desire or interest.

But... how?

No explanation to this so-called 'binding problem' is given.

Most of the other 'theories' attempting to explain the dynamic binding taking place in real time, in the complex process of consciousness, have concentrated on the human visual system. The best known is the one proposed by Crick and Koch, where stereotaxic studies of the cat's visual cortex revealed oscillations in the 35-70 hertz range, all firing in 'synchrony'. They suggested that "this synchronized firing, on or near the beat of a 'gamma oscillation' (35-70 hertz), might be the neural correlate of visual awareness."

Subsequent research in other animal species, including humans, has demonstrated that neuronal synchrony may be related to perceptual integration, the construction of coherent representations, attentional selection and awareness. Despite all the exciting advances in systems neuroscience and with the insight that many of our cognitive capacities, so heavily a part of our conscious experience, appear to be built-in domain-specific operations, we think we are a unified conscious agent with a past, a present and a future.

These domain-specific or modular systems are fully capable of producing behaviors, mood changes and cognitive activity. So with all this independent activity, what allows for this sense of conscious unity that we can "self"?

It turns out that we, as humans, have a specialized system to carry out this interpretive synthesis and it is located in the left hemisphere. Known as the interpreter by Gazzaniga and Ledoux, its discoverers, this system seeks explanations for how contiguous events relate to one another. It operates on other adaptations built into our brains. The adaptations are most likely cortically based but they work largely outside of conscious awareness, as do most of our mental activities.

Gazzaniga and associates wanted to know whether the emotional response to stimuli presented to one-half of a split-brain patient would affect the other half. They found that the emotional valence of the stimulus clearly crossed over from the right to the left hemisphere. The left remained unaware of the content that produced the emotional change, but it interpreted and experienced the emotion.

For example, if the command "walk" is flashed to the right half, the patient typically stands up and heads for the door. When asked where he is going, the patient shrugs and says, (using the left half to analyze and speak) "Oh, to the vending machine for a soda."

The brain's modular organization has now been well established. The functioning modules do have some kind of physical instantiation, but the brain scientists cannot yet specify the nature of the neural networks. However, what is clear is that these networks operate mainly outside the realm of awareness and announce their computational products to executive systems that mediate behavior or cognitive states.

Catching up with all of this parallel and constant activity appears to be the responsibility of the left hemisphere's interpreter module. The interpreter is a system of primary importance to the human brain: It allows for the formation of beliefs, which in turn are mental constructs that free us from simply responding to stimulus-response aspects of daily life.

With this view, it becomes evident that what we mean by consciousness is how we *feel* about our specialized capacities. Our consciousness is essentially an inferential system that collates all sorts of mental activity and assigns feelings to them. It reflects the *affective* component of specialized systems that have evolved through the intricate process of natural selection to enable human cognitive processes and become personalized "qualia".

The Search for 'Qualia'

Much of our understanding of the animal CNS (Central Nervous System) leads us to the classic picture in which neurons, consisting of a cell body housing a nucleus, extend out into a long un-branched axon at one end and a profusely branched dendrite at the other. The dendrites receive stimuli and conduct impulses generated by those stimuli toward the cell body. There is some evidence of 'dentritic processing' taking place. The cell body then sends out a 'graded response' out through the axon to the specific tissue for execution of the proper action.

Communication from neuron to neuron occurs at the synapse, where a terminal branch of the axon of one neuron makes contact with the cell body, dendrites or axon of another neuron. This communication can occur through electrical or chemical synapses. The electrical synapses consist of low-resistance connections between the membranes of two neurons where a change in potential in a pre-synaptic neuron transmits to a post-synaptic one with little attenuation. Electrical synapses are ubiquitous in the invertebrate and lower-vertebrate nervous system and at some sites in the mammalian nervous system.

The chemical synapses are the predominant type of inter-neuronal communication in the mammalian brain. Action potentials in the pre-synaptic neuron cause the release of neurotransmitters or neuro-modulators from synaptic vesicles. These 'chemical messengers' traverse the synaptic clefts and mediate excitatory or inhibitory responses on the post-synaptic membranes.

As is evident from the above description, there is a distinct 'qualitative' difference between the 'simple' electrical synapses found in the 'lower' life forms and the more complex synaptic terminals of 'higher' ones. The neurons connect to each other locally to form a dense network in portions of the brain called *gray* matter; they communicate over longer distances via fiber tracts called *white* matter.

The cortex itself is a six-layered structure with various connection patterns in each layer. There is an enormous amount of variability and uniqueness in each individual brain, which provides the organism with an organizing principle for the proper assessment of the environment it, is in. This perceptual categorization takes place by means of so-called *global mappings* that connect various modal maps stored in its memory.

The cortex subdivides into regions that mediate different sensory modalities, such as hearing, touch and sight. There are other cortical regions dedicated to motor functions that ultimately drive our muscles. Beyond the sensorimotor portions concerned with gathering information about the outside environment and modifying the internal one to meet those demands, there are regions of the brain such as the frontal, parietal and temporal 'lobes' that 'talk' to each other and maintain homeostasis in the physical body.

Many neurologists now believe that the *modulatory* neurons confer some permanent structural change on the brain cells that they contact. This *change* may constitute the same fundamental mechanism of learning and memory at all levels of the animal kingdom. Memory is a central component of the brain mechanisms that mediate an SOC.

It is commonly assumed that memory involves the inscription and subsequent storage in so-called 'association areas'. However, *what* is stored?

Is it an encoded message in some cryptic neuro-molecule that is yet to be discovered?

Or... Is it simply a complex jigsaw puzzle, hastily reconstructed from the coordinated input of disparate areas of the human cortex?

These queries point to the widespread assumption among the *laity* that what is stored in your 'head' is a long 'videotape', which has meticulously recorded every event of their lives.

The Edelman-Tononi team takes a different view. They shy away from depicting memory as the inscriptions on the *tabula rasa*. Instead, they describe memory as the ability of a dynamic system to repeat or suppress a mental or physical act if deemed inappropriate. They illustrate this novel and rather intriguing view of memory as similar to the melting and refreezing of glacial ice. Just as water undergoes multiple transition phases as the ambient temperature hovers around its freezing point, our memory has properties that allow perception to alter recall and recall to alter perception.

It has no fixed capacity limit since it actually generates *information* by 'constructing' it. It is robust, dynamic, associative and adaptive. It is one of the essential components of this complex biological process of Consciousness. By virtue of being 'creative' rather then merely replicative, it ultimately gives rise to 'Qualia', the so-called higher-order subjective responses to things we perceive. These when bound together into a *unitary* concept constitutes an SOC.

Primary consciousness arises as a result of circuitous interactions between brain areas mediating value-category memory stores and those 'association areas' of the cortex which derive perceptual precepts based on a weighted average of the incoming sensorimotor data. A consequence of such interactions is the 'construction' of a perceptual 'scene' out there and the ability to respond appropriately to it. This discriminatory capability within a unitary scene is often based on Qualia, the custom-made higher-order and privileged properties of consciousness in any given organism.

In humans, just as the separate snapshots in a film reel are translated into a smoothly flowing movie, the circuitous integration of neural input via numerous cortical areas, give rise to a unitary precept of Qualia. It cannot be divided into separate parts as it is experienced. Instead, the conscious 'scene' is unified and coherent. It is not possible, willfully or with even a high degree of attention to limit awareness to just one component of a scene to the exclusion of all others. Yet, myriad conscious states and scenes can be experienced sequentially with no subjective evidence of discontinuity or disruption. Consciousness itself is an *internally* constructed phenomenon.

In other words, although perceptual input is initially important, the integration of various areas and modalities in the cortex allows the individual to go beyond the information given. This going beyond, with the appearance of 'filling-in' and gestalt properties involving shifting dominances between cortical maps can be seen in various visual, auditory or somatosensory illusions to which all of us are prone. The same is true of the sense of time, of succession and of duration. The neural integration tends to combine concepts and precepts with its experiential memory stores to construct a coherent, self-consistent picture.

This 'phenomenal transform' of the neural input to the subjective concept of Qualia is one of the major origins of the subjective sense and in humans the notion of self-consciousness. Christof Koch in his book on *the Quest for Consciousness* theorizes that most people would reflexively assign consciousness to the top of the processing pyramid, which starts with the eyes, ears, nose and other sensors and ends with the 'conscious me' endpoint of all perception and memory.

In his opinion, this view is *false*; a mere 'cherished chimera'. Instead, he speculates that the neural correlates of consciousness (NCC), may reside in a so-called cognitive architecture straddling a representation of physical objects and events and an inner, hidden world of thoughts and concepts. He invokes Ray Jackendoff's analysis, which assumes a tripartite division of the mind-body into the physical brain, the computational mind and the phenomenological mind.

In his book *Consciousness and the Computational Mind*, Jackendoff defends a so-called *intermediate-level theory* of consciousness. He argues that even though common sense suggests that awareness and thought are inseparable and that introspection reveals the contents of the mind, both these beliefs are untrue. According to him, thinking i.e. the manipulation of concepts, sensory data or more abstract patterns, is largely *not* conscious.

What *is* conscious about thoughts, are images, tones, silent speech and to a lesser degree, other bodily feelings associated with *intermediate-level* sensory representations. Neither the process of thought nor its content is knowable by consciousness. In other words, you are not directly conscious of your inner world, although you have the persistent *illusion* that you are!

Koch elaborates: "you are only conscious then of representations of external objects (including your own body) or internal events by proxy. You are not directly conscious of something in the world, say a chair, but only of its visual and tactile representation in the cortex. The chair is out there; your only direct knowledge of it is derived from explicit but intermediate representations of your senses in your brain that leave out many fine details...

Likewise, recalled or imagined things are, mapped onto visual, olfactory, gustatory, vestibular, tactile and proprioceptive representations. A subset of these, the NCC, is experienced as *Qualia*. These involve one or more dominant coalitions stretching between cortical regions in the back and more frontal ones."

Whether the *Qualia* associated with these feelings, more diffuse and less detailed than sensory percepts, exist in their own right or are mixtures or modifications of various bodily sensations, is unclear.

Some researchers, Dennett for example, assert that sentient experiences or qualia are a cognitive *illusion* (there's that word again). Once we have isolated the computational and neurological correlates of access-consciousness, there is nothing left to explain? He feels that it is irrational to insist that qualia remain unexplained even after all its manifestations have been accounted for.

To him this is like insisting that *wetness* remains unexplained after all the manifestations of the water molecule have been described in detail. Well, as a sentient human, the unexplained quality of wetness does leave behind a feeling of dissatisfaction for me. It implies that just because we do not yet have a scientific explanation of cognitive perception, it does not exist.

In my opinion, Dennett is trying to banish this phenomenon from discourse by invoking the doctrine of logical positivism i.e. if a statement cannot be scientifically verified, it is essentially meaningless. He is really not explaining qualia as much as explaining it away.

Cybernetics and Neurophysiology

The advent of cybernetics into neurophysiology (1948), with its mathematical mind-set, produced a ripple effect in the scientific circles. The publication of Prof. Wiener's book on cybernetics, was soon followed by the growing awareness that both the 'computing machines' and the nervous system could be analyzed and described in terms of communication and control as they were in fact, both, information processing systems.

Dr. Wiener had argued on several occasions that the 'particles' in matter, machines and biological tissues were all equally comparable. Initially, his main concern was a study of the various types of neuro-physiological phenomena when different control mechanisms were applied to the human brain.

His earlier thoughts had centered on the evaluation of cortical alpha rhythms noticed on the EEGs. According to him, these types of 'constant' rhythms must have been the product of millions of cortical neurons undergoing a 'high degree of synchronization'. He saw that a control mechanism was at work here, quite separate from the all-or-nothing 'law' of evoked potentials.

His reasoning being that whereas the all-or-nothing principle applied for the long, myelinated nerve fibers in the CNS, some other mechanism must be responsible for the 'local' effects found in the shorter 'association' fibers i.e. a full 'spike' could not possibly develop over such short fibers.

In his words: "My idea is that we do have radiation within the nervous system but for a very short range. What you will ultimately get is a 'radiant' phenomenon, which is of such short weak range that you do not get it to the outside... Alpha rhythms can be thought of as the *synchronization* of the micro-radiation of individual neurons."

The concept seemed to fit with quantum analysis where wave functions characterized vibrating particles. The next step was to show how these specific micro-radiations come about.

Nucleic acid complexes were implicated.

It was felt that this 'synchronization' phenomenon was rooted in 'crystalline vibrations' being produced at a 'high frequency', which further led to the generated 'resonance' effect. Nucleic acid complexes were believed at that time to be the basis of memory in brain tissue. This reasoning followed from the 'fact' that all crystalline structures have specific spectrums of vibrations and therefore could 'answer' the specificity of the memory storage process.

Another 'pet theory' of Dr. Wiener was what he called a 'rhythmic system'. By this, he meant that randomly distributed particles or objects in a state of rhythmic oscillation could affect one another through interactions between them. He attributed this to a sort of a non-linear 'feed-back of information' and a kind of 'pooling-effect'. He found it in electrical generators, computers and also in biological organisms.

He had noticed that on warm pleasant evenings, all the frogs would croak in unison and all fireflies would flicker together.

The point Wiener was making was that here was an example of a 'control mechanism' in the behavior between animals. The frogs and fireflies, even though possessing individual 'natural rhythms' of either croaking or flickering, when taken as a group, tended to produce one synchronized rhythm.

Interestingly, this phenomenon is also observed in co-eds that dorm together. Most end up 'coordinating' their menses to cluster around the same time each month. Here again was this pooling-effect, this 'control mechanism' where animals responded to each other as if 'in unison'.

Gerald Edelman of the Scripps Research Institute, La Jolla, California and his colleague, Giulio Tononi, now at the University of Wisconsin, stress such a 'global' aspect of consciousness. They argue that the large number of potential states accessible to a conscious mind necessitates the tight interaction of very large neuronal assemblies spanning vast areas of the brain.

Their hypothesis has two basic tenets:

One, a select group of neurons can contribute directly to conscious experience only if it is a part of a distributed functional cluster that through 'reentrant' interactions in the thalamo-cortical system, achieves high integration in milliseconds and

Two, in order to sustain conscious experience, it is essential that this functional cluster be highly differentiated, as indicated by higher values of complexity.

They call this 'functional cluster of integrated neurons' a *dynamic core* in order to emphasize both its integration and it's constantly changing composition. They are quick to point out that this 'dynamic core' is a 'process', rather than a thing or location in the brain. Furthermore, since participation in the dynamic core depends on the rapidly shifting functional connectivity among groups of neurons, rather than on anatomical proximity, the actual composition of the core can sometimes transcend the traditional anatomical boundaries.

They assert that the exact composition of the core related to particular conscious states varies significantly from person to person. Each mind, according to them, is unique, not fully exhaustible by scientific means, and definitely not a machine. Conscious thought, to them, is a set of relations with a meaning that goes beyond just energy or matter (although it involves both).

One interesting point they bring up when asked about the 'mind', which gives rise to a thought, is that the mind is both material and 'meaningful' i.e. there is a material basis for the mind as a tangible 'set' of relationships. The activity of your brain and all its mechanisms results in an entity, which is concerned with the processes of meaning. There is a realm created by the physical order of the brain, the body and the social world to which 'meaning' is consciously given.

This 'meaning' is essential to both our description of the world around us and to our scientific understanding of it. According to Edelman-Tononi, it is the amazingly complex 'material structures' of the nervous system and body give rise to the dynamic mental processes and to meaning. They insist that nothing else needs to be assumed or invoked: neither other worlds, nor spirits, nor remarkable forces that remain unplumbed. There are no completely separate domains of matter and mind and no grounds for Dualism.

Being human in mind and brain appears clearly to be the result of an evolutionary process. They call it Neural Darwinism and profess that each individual's brain is continually changing. These variations extend over all levels of brain organization, from biochemistry to gross morphology and the strengths of myriad synapses undergo constant alteration by the individual's life experiences.

To uncover the neural mechanisms of consciousness, it is useful to keep in mind the distinction between primary and higher-order consciousness. Primary consciousness occurs in animals with certain brain structures similar to ours. They are able to construct a mental scene but with limited semantic or symbolic capabilities and no true language. Higher-order consciousness comes with a sense of Self and the ability in the waking state to explicitly construct past and future scenes. It requires, at the minimum, a semantic capability and in its most developed form, a robust linguistic capability.

Edelman-Tononi propose that the primary consciousness emerged in evolution when, through the appearance of new circuits mediating reentry, posterior areas of the brain that are involved in perceptual categorization were dynamically linked to the anterior ones responsible for mediating a value-based memory. They think that with such means in place, an animal would be able to build a remembered present – a scene that adaptively links immediate or imagined contingencies to that animal's prior history of value-driven behavior.

This model assumes that during evolution, the cortical systems leading to perceptual categorization were already in place before primary consciousness debuted. Then with the further development of secondary cortical areas and the various cortical 'appendages', such as the basal ganglia, conceptual memory systems gradually emerged. This, in turn, heralded a massively reentrant connectivity between the multi-modal cortical areas capable of carrying out perceptual categorization and the areas responsible for a value-category memory.

Edelman-Tononi define reentry as a process of ongoing parallel and recursive signaling between separate brain maps along massively parallel anatomical connections, most of which are reciprocal. It alters and amenable to alteration by the activity of the target areas it interconnects. It is critical to a variety of neural processes ranging from perceptual categorization and motor coordination to consciousness itself.

It also assures the integration that is essential to the creation of a scene in primary consciousness leading to a coherent output. This takes place through establishing short-term temporal correlations and synchrony among the activities of widely spaced neuronal groups, enabling them to fire simultaneously. This so-called *binding* principle then repeats across many levels of brain organization and seems to play a key role in mediating consciousness.

However, all the theories of neural binding considered so far, *assume* that the final result is not only unified conscious percepts but some kind of overall integration or synchrony in a unified 'field' of experience.

Semir Zeki, a neurobiologist at the University College of London, England, questions this view. According to him, there are as many 'micro-consciousnesses' as there are processing nodes in a system. He describes the primate visual system as consisting of many separate, specialized systems, working in *parallel*, each of which is autonomous and reaches a perceptual endpoint at a different time.

This inherent *multiplicity* of connections and the fact that no node is a recipient only implies that "there is no terminal station in the cortex." Some attributes are perceived before others, even though we may not be aware of this perceptual *asynchrony*. In Zeki's view, no *final* integrator is really needed in the brain. Each of the separate cortical systems involved has its own conscious correlate.

Consciousness and Altered States

The term, Consciousness, includes two distinct concepts: the actual state of consciousness i.e. whether the individual animal or human is awake, drowsy or asleep, and the second concept of the conscious experience, which refers to cognitive perception or 'awareness' i.e. what the individual animal or human is 'thinking' and 'doing' during this state.

The state of consciousness can be easily monitored by observation and testing. It is usually depicted by the EEG scan, which records the pattern of brain activity through electrodes attached at various locations on the scalp.

The EEG, technically known as the electro-encephalogram, is about a hundred times smaller than the amplitude of an evoked potential and its frequency may vary between 3 to 40 Hz. Each EEG pattern is the result of varying degrees of intermittent synchronization of membrane potential changes in groups of neurons, located in the cerebral cortex. These *graded* synaptic potentials rather than action potentials manifest more or less synchronous electrical fluctuations, analogous to the 'pooling-effect' mentioned earlier by Dr. Wiener.

The intralaminar and midline nuclei of the thalamus act as 'pacemaker' or rhythm generators, each of which projects to and influences the activity of a specific region of the cortex. These nuclei of the dorsal thalamus constitute an unexplored and poorly understood region.

Phylogenetically, these nuclei are older than the specific relay nuclei, which compose a large part of the human thalamus. Most of them have no cortical projections, though they appear to have established connections with other thalamic nuclei and the Striatum. Afferent projections to parts of the intralaminar nuclei derive from the spinal cord, the reticular formation, the cerebellum, the globus pallidus and broad cortical areas.

Stimulation of the ascending RAS, results in a generalized behavioral arousal of the animal. This arousal response is mediated, at least in part, by the intralaminar nuclei. Physiological studies suggest that impulses producing these changes in cortical activity reach the cortex via a diffuse, non-specific thalamic projection system.

Studies utilizing retrograde axonal transport of the enzyme, horseradish peroxidase, indicate that these projections are collaterals of fibers from the intralaminar thalamic nuclei, the principal ones of which terminate in the Neostriatum.

Stimulation of the so-called nonspecific thalamic nuclei and the basal diencephalic region through electrode implants produce widespread and pronounced effects on the EEG of the animal under study. The nonspecific thalamic nuclei include the intralaminar, the midline and the VA nucleus of the ventral tier.

Repetitive stimulation is seen to alter spontaneous electro-cortical activity over large areas of the brain and, under certain conditions, actually resets the frequency of the brainwaves by eliciting responses that are time-locked to the thalamic stimulus. The most characteristic effect observed during such sessions is the *recruiting* response.

Here, when the frequency of the stimulation is in the range of 6 to 12 Hz, rapidly increase, by the fourth to sixth stimulus, to a max of 40 Hz and then seem to taper off over a wide area of the cortex. This seems to be under the 'control' of the ascending reticular formation, as they cease firing upon stimulation of the bulbar RF.

In all fairness, no one knows what function, if any, this pattern of electro-cortical activity serves in the brain's task of information processing. We do not know whether these electric waves actually influence brain activity or that they just represent an epi-phenomenon i.e. a condition arising along with an event but not causally related to it. For example, the sound of a golf-ball striking the club: it results from the impact but really does not ensure a hole-in-one!

The world of science has long been aware that altered states of consciousness do exist, or can be induced not only by the classical *shamanic* and *yogic* practices, but also by the use of psychedelic drugs. The important fact to be noted here is that whatever the specific nature of the altered SOC, they always tend to make our subtle connections to each other and to our environment, more evident.

The 'mental' traffic between our interconnected minds and the rest of humanity is constant and seems to flow in both directions. We send our thought-impressions out to others who, in turn, signal back their reply. Every transaction leaves a subtle but indelible trace on the *Akashic* record.

Scientists have found that most animals, including humans, react to electro-magnetic signals and disturbances with a variety of symptoms. It appears that quasi-static and low frequency electro-magnetic 'fields' seem to link up directly with electro-magnetic 'codes', which were recently discovered in the information transfer and storage mechanisms of our CNS.

Further, some studies indicate that SpaceTime transcending information reaches our 'mind' when we enter a free ranging altered SOC, such as the white-dream state that is occurs between wakefulness and sleep. During this *hypnogogic* state, some 'primitive' cultures are able to access these realms quite readily and often.

In many parts of the world, meditation-adepts are able to combine devotional chanting, deep rhythmic breathing, hypnotic drumming, dancing and even specific forms of pain to induce these altered SOCs: For example, the !Kung bushmen of the Kalahari, certain native cultures of Africa and pre-Columbian America have used them in shamanic procedures, healing ceremonies and various rites-of-passage episodes.

The high cultures of Asia made use of them in numerous systems of *Raja Yoga*, *Vipassana* or *Zen* Buddhism; the ancient Egyptians used them in the Temple initiations of *Isis* and *Osiris*; the classical Greeks used them in *Bacchanalia*, the rites of *Attis* and *Adonis* and in the famous *Eleusian* mysteries.

Drugs and Altered States

Psychoactive drugs are all those pharmaceuticals or generic agents that affect mental function or the prevailing SOC. In some form or another, they are ubiquitous in modern society and human beings show a unique propensity to indulge in their use.

According to Atkins et al., "an altered state of consciousness exists whenever there is a change from an ordinary pattern of mental functioning to a state that *seems* different to the person experiencing the change." Even though this definition seems to capture the basic idea of what an altered state could be, by promoting more of a 'subjective' outlook, it raises many critical issues.

For example, how does one determine for sure if the induced state is *uniform* throughout the general population i.e. how can we tell if your 'trip' is anything like mine?

In addition, are any of these drug-induced states truly 'mind-blowing' spiritual experiences or just idle ramblings of a 'poisoned' *psyche?*

Psychoactive drugs come in all flavors and are broadly classified into several major groups like stimulants (uppers), depressants (downers), narcotics, anti-psychotics, anesthetics, anti-depressants and psychedelics. Of these, the last group is the most controversial and includes DMT (dimethyltryptamine, an active ingredient of *ayahuasca*), psilocybin (found in 'shrooms'), and mescaline (derived from the *peyote* cactus).

Many other synthetic hallucinogens or 'designer drugs' like LSD, numerous phenethylamines and tryptamine analogs induce varying effects over disparate time courses. The much maligned and disparaged, *cannabis*, used by the 'flower generation' of yore also falls into this category. With its

210

complex and varying mixture of psychoactives, *cannabis* nicely contrasts the relatively benign naturally occurring ones like *ayahuasca*, mescaline and psilocybin versus the starker effects of the so-called 'designer drugs' of the twenty-first century.

Even though users report many indescribable effects that vary in degree with the amount ingested or inhaled, scientific studies in various laboratories around the world show a mish-mash of effects on cognitive and emotional functions. However, psychedelics have changed many lives and encouraged users to "see things as they really are". However, are these drug-induced SOCs valid 'spiritual experiences' or just confabulations of a poisoned consciousness?

The presence of disparate altered states that are not merely transient, as in drug-induced, but which profoundly affect changes in the inductee's life occur as so-called 'exceptional human experiences' (EHEs). These encompass psychic visions, lucid dreams, 'out-of-body experiences' (OBEs), 'near-death experiences' (NDEs) or various other 'mystical'/ spiritual experiences.

While undergoing such episodes, the ordinary sense of a conscious Self, seems to undergo a dramatic disruption. The person emerges quite *transformed*; often with a different outlook on life, a changed belief system and a reduced fear of death. Some of these experiences prompt paranormal or supernatural claims. Others may be taken as evidence for the existence of an omnipotent Deity, souls, spirits or life after death. What they surely do is raise numerous questions in the scientific world.

Are any of these claims valid? Is there a common thread running through these mystical experiences or are they just a loose collection of unrelated oddities?

Certain psychoanalytic theories describe the OBE as a dramatization of the fear of death, which Jung saw as part of the process of individuation. They find that OBE's tend to predominate when there is a *mismatch* between the sensory input to the brain and the individual's body image. When a weak electric current was passed via a microelectrode into the right angular gyrus of the temporal lobe, the patient reported a 'sinking' or 'floating' sensation that increased with current intensity.

She also reported on various body image *distortions* during the stimulation and felt like she was *detached* from her physical body and observing everything being done to her from the ceiling. Interestingly enough, epileptic patients with lesions of the temporal lobe report more such OBE experiences.

Near-death experiences, on the other hand, are commonly taken to be proof-positive of the existence of "a higher spiritual world", or a soul that can survive death by leaving the body. An alternative, more *naturalistic* approach to understanding this process of NDE, known as the "dying brain hypothesis", was introduced in 1993 by Susan Blackmore of Oxford University. She mentions that severe stress, extreme fear and high degrees of cerebral anoxia all cause cortical disinhibition and spasmodic brain activity.

Bright images of lights and tunnels are frequently caused by disinhibition in the visual cortex and the so-called 'life reviews' reported by accident victims can be induced by stimulation of the temporal lobe. The positive emotions and apparent lack of pain were attributed to the action of endorphins, encephalins or endogenous opiates released under extreme stress.

These visions of other worlds and spiritual beings may be real glimpses into the *Void*, except for the intriguing cultural bias that seems to exude from the description of such episodes. For example, Hindus relate *darshans* of their own deities decked out in fine regalia, the Parsees describe visions of *Ahura Mazda*, and Christians greet Jesus in a restored Garden of Eden, or by the pearly gates, with evidence of bloody stigmata in plain sight and the Muslims describe lucid visions of vestal virgins cavorting in a paradisiacal oasis.

Mystical experiences are rather diverse and almost impossible to define in succinct terms. In William James' opinion, the bottom line is, "the whole concern of both morality and religion is the manner of our acceptance of the universe". He proposed *four* hallmarks of a mystical experience. *Ineffability* (the inability to describe it in words or successfully impart its emotional content to others), *transience* (tendency to not last too long), passivity (the mystic feels that a 'higher force' is in total control) and possessing a so-called '*noetic*' quality, a term that James coined to describe a superior state of knowledge, insight or illumination.

Deep mystical experiences seem to transcend narrow parochial religious views. In the Essentials of Mysticism, Evelyn Underhill sought to 'disentangle the facts from ancient formulae used to express them'. She defined the essence of mysticism as the clear conviction of a living god in unity with the personal self. Underhill specifically rejected paranormal claims as missing the point. Even Buddhist initiates are taught to ignore visions, miracles and faith healing. "They are no better than dreams which vanish forever on awakening".

Dismissing such reports/experiences as fabrications or wish fulfillment, even though easy, is unreasonable. The similarities observed across the ages and diverse cultures along with the inherent reliability of ones that underwent meticulous monitoring in various labs around the world seem to suggest that these may have something interesting to teach us about the process of death and our human *psyche*.

When viewed dispassionately they seem to push the limits of the mind-brain relationship as understood by our current state of comprehension and compel us to develop a newer, broader, more encompassing 'science' of consciousness.

Epilogue

The human lineage originated well over four *million* years ago in an evolutionary event that resulted in a dramatic shrinkage of habitable woodlands. This global catastrophe, heralding the onset of the so-called Ice Ages, induced the early humans dwelling in the African continent to adapt quickly or perish. As a result, the *hominids* (ancestral humans) began to acquire physical characteristics that made them neither as talented up in the trees as the great apes nor as facile on *terra firma* as modern humans.

Over the next million years, our ancestors and their upright relatives gradually adapted to the tumultuous environment in which they found themselves and began to flourish. They also continued to "morph" into numerous sub-species that occupied a continuum of bipedal physiologies. However, it was not until the next major climatic crisis that the early *hominids* initiated the routine use of stone tools, which transformed them from a prey item on the African savanna into a capable and deviously innovative scavenger-forager.

Cognitively speaking, the first toolmakers had moved far beyond the pale of other *hominid* competitors. They displayed a keen insight into the properties of stone and how it could be fractured into a handy cutting instrument. Utilizing this basic tool to skin and quarter animal carcasses, the early *Homo* succeeded in expanding his food choices. He was able to incorporate nutritious animal meats in his daily menu.

The transformation was a profound one. Here, finally, was a scrawny bipedal hominid that was completely at home in open country despite the many dangers it posed for a creature that lacked the hooks and claws of other predators. Instead of helplessly accepting the incapacitating onslaughts of the aggressive beasts, Homo could fend them off with a few jabs of his trusty weapons.

However, a few hundred millennia elapsed before the early *Homo* lineage introduced any detectable cultural innovation that focused not merely on the sharpness of the cutting tool but on its portability. For, in order to make a carefully honed axe, one not only had to understand the cleaving pattern and hardness of various rocks but conceptualize the fabrication process.

Our cognitive ability as full-fledged *Homo sapiens sapiens* emerged some 150,000 years ago in the Great Rift Valley of Eastern Africa via the culling process of natural selection. Its main purpose back then was to resolve problems that were life threatening to our early human ancestors. The challenge facing them was not to discover the *correct* solution or explanation of *how* things happen out there in the real world but to arrive at a plausible reason for that particular occurrence or natural phenomena.

We can well imagine fellow creatures with lesser cognitive abilities, like our pets that may excel in numerous situations but are quite dependent on their human benefactors for food and shelter. Just as your trained parrot can repeat phrases without really understanding their meaning, why should we be expected to comprehend all natural mysteries and grasp all truths related to free will and sentience?

As Steven Pinker observes in *How the Mind Works*, we should be thankful that the problems of science are close enough in structure to the daily problems of our foraging ancestors that we have made the progress that we have in the span of a few millennia. We have invented technologies that have enhanced all our senses a thousand-fold, we live in shelters that protect us from the vagaries of natural forces, we can travel around the world in a few days, observe our disorderly brethren from miles away, destroy them all if we so choose with the touch of a button or even land and explore other terrestrial bodies of the solar system.

Human sentience is not simply a combination of discrete brain events or behavioral states. The sense of self is not a combination of body parts or bits of information "pieced" together into a unitary concept. Free will is not a causal chain of events or the mental cogitations of a cortical module in the prefrontal lobe. Alas, the brain scientists can no longer invoke some so-called "interpreter" or master puppeteer, neatly ensconced within the forebrain that manipulates the self through various lifestyles.

Thoughts and thinking are no longer ghostly enigmas but mechanistic processes that are amenable to scientific study. The immense computational power of human thought and inventiveness has been put to good use in the marvelous applications of high technology found all around us today.

However, the problem of explaining how the brain enables human conscious experience still remains a deep mystery to most neuroscientists. From the foregoing text, it is quite obvious that we have accumulated vast amounts of information on how various regions of the brain are responsible for mental and perceptual activities. It is also evident that we may never figure out why some kinds of information processing in the brain gives rise to sentient experience instead of just input and output.

We may speculate that the proverbial lab rat laboring to get to the piece of cheese at the end of the maze was aided by some divine entity to reward its efforts. In a similar way, humans might invent all kinds of *cockamamie* theories about our place in this world and how we all got here in the first place. We would invoke the powers of this Almighty, invent religion and philosophy and go round and round pontificating about these questions for thousands of years with no real progress or true answers to this dilemma.

However, as scientists, we know that there are a myriad of problems not conducive to a simple explanation that would satisfy all aspects of human cognition. Issues of access, self-knowledge, attention, perception and feelings of sentience are all addressable through the avid pursuit of science. Current avenues of research and mapping techniques are illuminating these issues and shedding a bright light on the study of conscious experience, key to understanding the workings of the human mind.

Bibliography

The Central Nervous System, Structure & Function, 3rd edition: Per Brodal

Cognitive Neuroscience: The Biology of the Mind; Gazzaniga, Ivry and Mangun

The Quest for Consciousness: Christof Koch

How the Mind Works: Steven Pinker

The Birth of the Mind: Gary Marcus

Mind Wide Open: Steven Johnson

Binocular Vision: R.W. Reading

Adapting Minds: David J. Buller

A Universe of Consciousness: Gerald Edelman & Giulio Tononi

Wider than the Sky: Gerald Edelman

Shadows of the Mind: Roger Penrose

Physiology of the Eye: Adler

Consciousness: An Introduction; Susan Blackmore

The Spiritual Universe: Fred Alan Wolf

Mysteries of the Mind: Restak

Vital Dust: Christian de Duve

The World of the Cell: Becker, Kleinsmith & Hardin

Mind: John Searle

Cybernetics of the Nervous System: Norbert Wiener

Buddha & His Teachings: Berchol & Kohn

The Bhagavad Gita: Paramahansa Yogananda

www.ingramcontent.com/pod-product-compliance
Lightning Source LLC
Chambersburg PA
CBHW081112170526
45165CB00008B/2419